PRAISE
DYNAMIC BALANCE

"*Dynamic Balance* demystifies the practical wisdom of traditional Chinese medicine applied to training and recovery. Armed with this perspective on balance, athletes can reap greater longevity and higher performance. Reading this book has reaffirmed my respect for the complex and resilient human body, mind, and spirit and the system created to help us understand it."

—AMY ACUFF, five-time US Olympian,
Track and Field—High Jump

"In this innovative collaboration, Andy and Stella travel between concepts of conventional western and Chinese medicine. This book is a delightful guide full of important information for coaches and athletes who want to take their performance to the next level."

—DR. EDUARDO SANTOS, Medical Director,
Shanghai Port Football Club

"*Dynamic Balance* is an exceptional text on leveraging Traditional Chinese Medicine to reach optimal health and performance. Author Andy Chan uses his years of experience in exercise science to show readers how Traditional Chinese Medicine can serve as a great complement to current exercise training models. He and coauthor Dr. Stella Wong lay out a practical and compelling case on why Traditional Chinese Medicine is key to establishing and maintaining Dynamic Balance. I highly recommend this text to exercise professionals, students, athletes, and fitness enthusiasts who seek a plan for optimal balance in fitness, lifestyle, and health."

—RONALD WAGNER, PhD, ATC, CES, PES,
CEO, Relearnit, Inc.

DYNAMIC BALANCE

Integrating Principles
of Traditional Chinese Medicine
into Strength and Conditioning

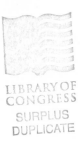

Tsz Chiu Chan, MS, CSCS
and Yat Kwan Wong, PhD

RIVER GROVE
BOOKS

This book is intended as a reference volume only, not as a medical manual. The information given here is designed to help you make informed decisions about your health. It is not intended as a substitute for any treatment that may have been prescribed by your doctor. If you suspect that you have a medical problem, you should seek competent medical help. You should not begin a new health regimen without first consulting a medical professional.

LCCN: 2021905790

Published by Well Spirit Press
Woodland Hills, CA
www.wellspiritcollective.com/wellspiritpress

Distributed by River Grove Books

Design and composition by Greenleaf Book Group
Cover design by Greenleaf Book Group and Mimi Bark

Images 696190536 and 696190502 ©iStockphoto.com/CasarsaGuru
Image 1139544143 ©iStockphoto.com/evgenyatamanenko
Lung Meridian art by Milos Vymazal
Photography by StevenC Photography

Publisher's Cataloging-in-Publication data is available.

Print ISBN: 978-1-7348601-2-2

eBook ISBN: 978-1-7348601-3-9

First Edition

*To all athletes
looking for an edge*

CONTENTS

Part 2: Seeking Sources of Imbalance and Fatigue

Part 3: Lifestyle Strategies for Dynamic Balance: Some Practical Pointers

Part 4: Developing Your Own Dynamic Balance Plan

Appendices

STRUGGLES WITH AN IMBALANCED APPROACH TO FITNESS

By Tsz Chiu "Andy" Chan

As one of the best soccer players from my high school in Conn-ecticut, I had my sights on playing at the collegiate level. Motivated by those around me, I started weightlifting around the eleventh grade. Like the majority of high schoolers, I just did whatever was deemed cool at the time—basically whatever the football and hockey guys did. The approach was haphazard and random—we didn't know what we were doing. Looking back, it is funny how my classmates and I thought we were so cool when we were yanking out those bicep curls.

Things got serious during the following summer vacation when I went back to Hong Kong. Determined to become a better athlete, I went to my local gym. When I talked with the enthusiastic membership sales-woman about my aspirations, she asked if she could take my basic body measurements, including height, weight, and body fat, as a baseline refer-ence. How could I say no to such a professional approach? She walked me to the InBody machine (a machine that analyzes body composition).

I still vividly remember the exchange that happened as I stepped on the scale, even though it was more than a decade ago.

The saleswoman grabbed on to my biceps and guided me with a gentle voice: "Let me help you to step on the machine, Andy."

Me: "Uh . . . " (What I was thinking was that the scale was about three inches off the ground, so surely I didn't need her help! But whatever . . .)

She then said in a demeaning tone: "Wow, you have got some girly arms. Even my arms are bigger than yours."

That statement ignited my innate passion and desire to prove her wrong. Not only did I join the gym, but my competitive nature also compelled me to hire a personal trainer, *right away*. I asked her to assign me to the biggest coach in that gym because I wanted to begin the sessions the following day. (Not so difficult to do business with a teenager, right? Turns out, many commercial gyms apply similar sorts of fear tactics to get innocent and gullible clients, like the teenage me, to sign up.)

Nonetheless, although I was somewhat scammed into the gym, I started working with a strict coach, thankfully. During the initial session, he asked about my strength training goals. I told him my ultimate goal was to become a better athlete (on my way to becoming a college soccer player!), but it would be nice if I could gain some muscles as well. He explained to me that muscular strength, power, and endurance could enhance my ability to perform different sports skills, so my two goals were related. This was music to my ears, because it meant that I could kill two birds with one stone.

Over the next three months of summer vacation, I worked the plan with my coach, who pushed me to my limits every single session. We trained about three to four times a week, on top of my soccer practices. In addition, I was instructed to follow his nutritional guidance. Because I was trying to gain muscle mass, I had to consume six or seven high-caloric meals per day full of carbohydrates and protein. I also had to incorporate mass-gainer protein shakes into my diet. To be honest, at times it felt as though I was constantly eating without a break. But I told myself it was necessary in order to become a college athlete.

After three months, I had gained about ten pounds, I went up a size in shirts, and my physique looked good, at least better than before. On the surface, one of my initial goals of becoming bigger was achieved.

Yet my performance did not match the same level of improvement. I noticed that my movements on the soccer field had started to become rigid, and my stamina had dropped. I had trouble sleeping at night. I was moody and easily agitated. Perhaps the worst side effect of all—from my teenage point of view—was the fact that my forehead and the sides of my face were filled with disgusting acne. Put simply, yes, I was getting bigger, but that was offset by my lack of sleep, mood swings, and a persistent negative body image.

I was frustrated. I wanted to become a better athlete. I got bigger, yet that did not translate to better performance.

So what went wrong?

Before answering that question, let me ask one of you. Do you see yourself or athletes you work with in my story? Most people I talk with have had similar experiences: The work they do to achieve one health or fitness goal puts something else in their life out of balance. Surely there must be a better approach.

What we now know is that all the physical and emotional challenges that we experience require management, and our work toward health and fitness must be woven into a more holistic approach of balancing everything that is going on in our lives. We need a *sustainable* strategy that can help us cope with the obstacles that we encounter throughout the day, as well as help us achieve our fitness and performance goals.

We also now know that overtraining—and, specifically, the lack of quality *recovery*—can lead to fatigue, nonspecific discomfort, and pain. To combat the fatigue and pain, some athletes are turning to stimulants and pharmaceuticals. While coffee and pills may relieve the symptoms of overtraining, those solutions are short-term and partial.

The pursuit of sustainability, recovery, and improved performance is why many athletes, coaches, and practitioners are now exploring natural ways to achieve better fitness, health, and lifestyle. And that's what this book is about.

TCM: A Missing Piece of the Puzzle

Let's start with the basics. Fitness warriors and their strength and conditioning coaches have two primary goals: (1) to improve athletic performance by improving athletes' power, strength, endurance, and speed and (2) to reduce the risk of athletic injuries.

To achieve these goals, we know that we must endure rigorous conditioning programs. But what does that mean? Historically, training sessions or practices in sports had to be "hard core," as the general conception was that intensive training sessions would strengthen athletes' mental and physical tolerance, thereby leading to better athletic performance.

In recent years, this mentality has evolved thanks to advances in sports science. Turns out, "no pain no gain" is an insidious mindset that moves athletes *further away* from excellence rather than bringing them closer to it.

Another factor is the recognition that each body responds to stress (physical or emotional) differently. Sure, there is a stage where the body overcomes the imposed demand or stress by becoming stronger, but there is also a stage where the athlete becomes exhausted and burned out.

The trick is to find a balance point between training load and recovery strategies so that an athlete can overcome stress and not hit exhaustion.

The search for a more balanced approach to fitness has led people like me to study traditional Chinese medicine (TCM).

Growing up in Hong Kong, I saw TCM clinics, pharmacies, and related companies everywhere. As I grew up, I'd see the Yin-Yang symbol being used in such diverse places as university clinics, temples, sporting facilities, and massage shops—and bizarrely, as the name of an American hip-hop duo. I never understood TCM concepts during childhood, other than the fact that it meant I had to drink some bitter herbal tea to stay healthy. That's why, even for kids like me who had some exposure to TCM growing up, the discipline always seemed more like myth than reality.

My interest in TCM changed a few years ago after I became a strength and conditioning coach. The image that piqued my curiosity in Oriental recovery methods was one from the 2016 Olympics, where Michael Phelps had some circular, dark, purply circles dotting his shoulders and back. For the next few months, the athletic community followed suit and began exploring the efficacy of the "cupping" treatment he received and other TCM procedures. Fast-forward to 2020, and images of athletes using Oriental recovery methods such as cupping, Gua Sha (scraping), and acupuncture are well circulated over social media and the internet. (You'll find more information on these topics in Chapter 3.4.)

What I and many others have come to realize is that the Chinese have been using TCM philosophies to maintain health, improve the quality of life, and treat sickness and injuries for thousands of years. TCM is a convergence, distillation, and collection of different doctrines, theories, and practices from nearly five millennia of application. They are focused on helping people live in balance with themselves and with nature.

To better understand specifically how athletes and strength and conditioning coaches can better utilize TCM concepts and methodologies, I was fortunate to be able to team up with my co-author, Dr. Yat Kwan "Stella" Wong, who is a licensed Chinese medicine practitioner. (In fact, Stella is a second-generation TCM practitioner.) Different from most conventional practitioners, she received a PhD in Chinese medicine from the University of Hong Kong after completing her undergraduate studies in Beijing, China. This meant that she was trained through both the Eastern and the Western education systems.

She understands the thought processes that we Western-educated people go through and can unpack the esoteric TCM language using simple analogies.

Mental and Physical Health

Stella is especially passionate in researching the effects of acupuncture in treating issues related to mental health. That's why, as you'll see later in this book, we focus on both the physical and mental side of fitness and health. Her insights in the psychological management chapters are invaluable to understanding how maintaining good health is not limited to the physical body but to the emotional aspects as well.

TCM CONTROVERSIES

Unfortunately, the only exposure that many people in the West have had to TCM is through some controversies that have made headlines. For example, after the World Health Organization included TCM diagnostic patterns in the 2019 revision of the International Classification of Diseases code—the global standard for diagnostic health—many Western-trained medical professionals objected because they feel that TCM lacks rigorous evidence. Some animal rights activists are also under the impression TCM fosters the widespread exploitation of endangered animals for their body parts.

We want to point out that TCM *is* time-tested (the earliest known written record of Chinese medicine, *The Yellow Emperor's Classic of Medicine*, was written in the third century BC). As we'll discuss in Part 3, the Eastern and Western approaches to "scientific proof" are still not quite in sync.

Furthermore, we, too, are concerned about endangered animals and plants. Dr. Lixing Lao—president of the Virginia University of Integrative

Medicine and the former director of the School of Chinese Medicine at the University of Hong Kong—has stated that 100% of Chinese medicine can be derived from plants. He also said that the use of endangered animals is indeed against the fundamental principle of TCM, in which harmony between humans and nature must be maintained.

So no matter your background or exposure to TCM, we ask that you keep an open mind as you go through this book. Try out some of the ideas to see if they help you achieve a more balanced lifestyle and better overall fitness.

Seeking Dynamic Balance

The title of this book, *Dynamic Balance*, comes from the TCM interest in what we in the West call *homeostasis*. The concept of homeostasis has been the cornerstone of human physiology ever since the term was coined by physiologist Walter Cannon in 1926. He built on the work of fellow physiologist Claude Bernard—who first spoke of the concept in 1865—and gave a new definition to the word that describes the self-regulating process that the body maintains while adjusting to changing conditions. That is, there is no fixed, single point of balance but rather a narrow range that is best for the health of our cells, tissues, and organs. Balance is therefore a matter of shifting within this narrow range—maintaining dynamic equilibrium—as conditions change within and outside our bodies.

That word *dynamic* is hugely overlooked in the fitness community. Our internal equilibrium is ever-changing with the environment, even if only slightly. Rather than approaching homeostasis like a binary *absolute* question—Are you balanced? Yes or no—remember that homeostasis is a dynamic range that the body maintains. Where your body is at this very moment will likely be slightly different from where it was a minute ago or where it will be a minute from now. Your ability to maintain *dynamic balance* will determine your overall health and fitness.

REACHING AND LOSING DYNAMIC BALANCE

The issue of how athletes can win and then lose dynamic balance is easily illustrated by the story of Bryan, a former client and now good friend of mine.

Bryan is about 5 feet, 5 inches tall. When we first began training, his weight was nearly two hundred pounds (32% body fat). During our initial meeting, he was timid and shy, with a slouching posture. He told me that his main priority was fat loss. Bryan and I trained three times a week, and he trained on his own for two days. Our sessions were typically quite intense, as I knew he generally would not push himself as much without the supervision of a coach. (This is true for many of us!)

My diet advice to Bryan was simple: Eat a bit of everything; avoid extreme diets. He was surprised when he first heard that. He had expected to be told to cut carbohydrates, sugar, and oily foods altogether. He came in with the expectation to suffer. But I insisted that this was not necessary because that sort of lifestyle is not sustainable.

After four months of training, Bryan's weight dropped to about 175 pounds (28% body fat). While these numbers are not as dramatic as the ones that are lauded in the media, we were on a great track because fat loss should be achieved gradually as the result of a sustainable lifestyle. Up until that point, he was satisfied with his progress. In fact, slouching and timid Bryan had turned into a smiling person brimming with confidence. He was so happy with his physique that he even started to love taking photos.

Then things took a downhill turn when Bryan became impatient. He wanted quicker results, a trap that we all invariably fall into more often than not.

At one point, he was doing five consecutive weekly sessions with me, Monday through Friday. I had explained to him that even though we were meeting five times per week, we had to alternate between different intensities because the body could not sustain consecutive days of high intensity without adequate rest and recovery. I pointed out that even the best players in the National Basketball Association will see a diminished performance after playing four games in five days. The body is just not built that way. It needs time to rest and recover.

In response, he told me that he was determined to find the best version of himself, and nothing would hold him back. (Similar to my personal gym story, ill-managed passion can inadvertently get us into trouble.) So for a few months, we did five sessions a week. I did my best to move him away from the extreme, but he refused. He wanted an intense session every single day. Outside of the training session, he decided to ignore my suggestions to steer away from extreme diets. He barely ate anything other than steamed chicken, boiled sweet potatoes, and steamed vegetables.

Bryan's lowest weight after that intense period of training was 145 pounds, just under 18% body fat.

Such an encouraging story . . . until it wasn't.

After the remarkable feat of getting to 145 pounds, Bryan went through challenges in his personal life. He became stressed out as he was starting a new business. Because he was stressed out, he lost control of his sleep and his diet. Even when he was eating "clean," he would still feel bloated. The number of gym sessions dropped from five times a week to three times a week, to once a week, to none. Bryan was stressed, hopeless, and defeated, and he gained twenty pounds in two months.

Bryan's dedication had driven his transformation, and he did, in fact, achieve his original goal of fat loss. But his approach had two serious flaws: First, he lacked a balance between his fitness approach and recovery, so his physical fitness got out of balance. And second, he lacked a *sustainable* life strategy that he could fall back on when life threw him a curveball, so he was unable to maintain his extreme diet and fitness routines.

Ultimately, Bryan fell into the same trap that I had fallen into and that captures many athletes: We treat our diet and fitness routines as something separate from the rest of our lives. We set specific fitness goals thinking that if we just strengthen a few specific muscles, we'll perform better.

That mentality is the exact opposite of what TCM teaches us. We need to switch our mentality so we look at our lifestyle and every component of our bodies as interconnected pieces. We have to define our own range of homeostasis in its broadest sense: how to structure our diets, fitness routines, and emotional health to maintain our own dynamic balance.

For many of us, including Bryan, 2020 was an unprecedented and challenging year. With mandatory gym closures and the seemingly never-ending lockdowns, it was important to have a strategy that could help us cope with the "new normal" (work from home, eat at home, stay at home). Through adopting the lifestyle strategies that are provided in this book, Bryan has stabilized his weight, because he learned that being in the extreme gets him nowhere. He is also optimistic and confident, because with gyms reopening and the economy starting to recover, he has introduced the gym sessions back into his daily routine.

Creating Your Own Dynamic Balance

Our ultimate goal for you is to appreciate the complexity of the human being from a broader perspective. We want you to look beyond the flexibility, strength, and cardiorespiratory metrics that are typically assessed on the field or at the gym. We want to introduce you to a framework that is based on reason and logic and a philosophy that has existed for centuries and is increasingly supported by modern scientific evidence.

Given the conceptual differences between Eastern and Western medicine, our book is designed to help you bridge the gap between the two philosophies. The book is written to be an educational journey in which you can actively participate:

- Part 1 provides a review of the basic principles of TCM and shows how they relate to health and fitness.

- Part 2 gives you the opportunity to complete a questionnaire to identify your body constitution type (according to TCM) and then reviews three common sources of imbalance linked to your constitution and steps you can take to counter imbalances.

- Part 3 describes proactive steps you can take to maintain optimal health and fitness, based on TCM principles.

- Part 4 provides the forms and instructions you need to start developing your personalized plan for dynamic balance.

The ultimate purpose of the book is to help strength and conditioning coaches, fitness instructors, and athletes better understand the core messages of traditional Chinese medicine, and we are really excited to go on this journey with you! Integrating TCM principles into a strength and conditioning program will help you and your athletes or your students perform better, recover better, and ultimately live healthier.

Let's get started.

PART 1

ESSENTIAL CHINESE

MEDICINE CONCEPTS

THE POETRY OF THE HUMAN BODY

As we mentioned in the Introduction, traditional Chinese medicine is a discipline that has been around for more than five millennia. But though it has been around far longer than Western medicine, knowledge about its concepts and practices is limited outside of China and other Asian countries. That's why the concepts and terminology used with TCM are culturally foreign to the Western world, and perhaps especially the athletic population.

What you should know up front is that TCM is a complex system of medicine based on the premise that good health relies on the maintenance of harmony and balance between the body and the surrounding environment—the dynamic balance that gave this book its title.

We don't expect you to become an expert in TCM overnight. But we hope the following chapters will give you a foundation that will help you better understand and apply the practices we will cover in Parts 2, 3, and 4. In the following chapters, we cover the major concepts of TCM and discuss their relationship to each other:

- Chapter 1.1: The Vital Substances of Life (Qi and Blood)
- Chapter 1.2: The Language of Balance and Harmony (Yin-Yang and Five Phases)
- Chapter 1.3: The Body Is Not a Machine (Zang-Fu and Meridians)
- Chapter 1.4: The Search for Smooth and Elegant Movements (Muscles and Fascia)

As you read through these chapters, you'll notice two key differences between the TCM concepts and Western medicine. First, all of the TCM concepts have both a physiological meaning and a philosophical meaning. Second, that philosophical meaning is tied to the fundamental belief that every part and function in the human body is part of an integrated whole. That is, in TCM the human body is not seen as just a set of physical structures. The body is instead defined by how all its components interact and how energy flows throughout the entire system.

In each chapter, we'll describe one of the concepts, discuss how it influences our understanding of how to achieve maximum health and performance, and talk about ways the concept should influence how you think about your own health and fitness.

THE VITAL SUBSTANCES OF LIFE (QI AND BLOOD)

In traditional Chinese medicine, Qi and blood are often grouped together in diagnosis or day-to-day conversations. Although they can be explained as individual concepts, they are intertwined together when describing life and circulation. Blood is easy to relate to—there is a visual and tactile connection to it, and maybe even an emotional connection. We can see it when we bleed. Qi is a little harder to grasp, as it is an abstract concept, but you can think of it as energy that fuels the body. To help you better understand how the terms Qi and blood were created and used, let's dive into the cultural perspective that TCM is embedded in.

Back in the day, scholars did not have the technology to conduct microscopy or randomized double-blind placebo-controlled studies, the gold standard in modern scientific research. Instead, through trial and error, the Chinese would observe patterns of nature and illness to look for connections. For this reason, many TCM concepts were expressed through abstract analogies. Let's begin with the breath of life.

Qi: The Breath of Life

You may think you know what Qi is because the term is used throughout popular culture in the West. In movies, Qi (pronounced "chee") is sometimes framed as a mystical energy that permeates the universe, something like the Force in *Star Wars*. Other times, it is treated as a myth. There have been countless debates and studies on the topic of Qi, many of which have only clouded the topic further.

The ancient Chinese viewed Qi as the beginning and fundamental substance of life. *The Yellow Emperor's Classic of Medicine*, a treatise on health and disease written around the third century BC, documented that everything found in nature is made of Qi. Plants have Qi, animals have Qi, even rocks have Qi. Humans, as part of this universe, are no exception. Substances and life are formed when Qi of different motions and properties integrate. Therefore, Qi is vital, as life is created from it! Simply put, because Qi is an energy that is constantly moving, *if Qi is moving smoothly, we flourish; if Qi stops moving, we die.*

Qi in Other Contexts

Though we are focusing on how Qi relates to the human body here, the word is not limited to its medical usage, as it is included in thousands of other Chinese words. For instance, *shí yóu qì* means petroleum gas, *qì fēn* means atmosphere, *qì něi* means discouraged, and *huàn qì* means to exchange gas/air or to ventilate. Although those four words have different meanings, they all describe some sort of energy—the energy that fuels cars, the energy of a concert, the energy of a person, and the act of breathing. Thousands of terms include the word Qi to create meaning. It is important to understand the context in which the word Qi is being used.

The meaning of Qi can change with context, sometimes referring to breath or air, sometimes to energy. To put it through the lens of human physiology, Qi is the word ancient Chinese physicians used to describe general functions of the human body. For us in the West, it's often helpful to think of Qi as the aspects of the human body that are invisible or imperceptible to the human eye.

A sensible thought at this stage might be that if we can somehow manage to balance our Qi, then we are all set. We'll learn as we go through the book that our Qi is constantly influenced by internal and external factors that are always changing. In other words, the body is *always* adjusting and adapting. Balanced Qi is a similar concept to homeostasis in human physiology. As such, the regulation of pH, body temperature, oxygen, hormones, neurotransmitters, electrochemical impulses, sensory receptors, and so on are all specific illustrations of Qi. To achieve good health, one's Qi must be balanced.

DIRECTIONS OF QI

Qi is like a vivid energy that moves in different directions. Balanced Qi implies that Qi is moving smoothly and unobstructed in all directions through the pathways of our bodies, thus maintaining health. Disruption in any direction would affect the transportation of Qi, thus yielding sickness. The movement of Qi can be broadly categorized into four basic directions: upward, downward, inward, and outward.

Every organ has a normal direction of flow that maintains normal function. The Qi of some organs (such as the stomach) flows downward, and the Qi of other organs (such as the spleen) flows upward. For organs like the liver, the movement of Qi is upward and outward.

How Directions of Qi Were Determined

Historically, the flow of Qi was deduced by observation. Ancient texts have documented that healthy stomach Qi flows downward because of its function—the stomach is in charge of digestion, and it passes digested food on to the next organ. Therefore, it is said to have a downward flow of Qi. The spleen, on the other hand, is an organ in charge of dispersing the essence of food to nourish other organs. Therefore, it needs an upward flow of Qi so that the essences can be distributed throughout the body.

Even if the concept of energy flow and its disruptions sounds odd to you, we bet that you have experienced it in your own life. For example, think of a recent incident that made you anxious. Perhaps it was that moment before a competition: Your heart was pounding, your face was turning red, and your muscles were tensing up. If not managed properly, that uneasy feeling might lead to headaches or fainting, which would hinder your performance. In severe cases, unpleasant emotions might even lead to a heart attack, although more research is needed to validate the connection between anxiety and heart attacks.

What is happening physiologically? From the Western perspective, stress activates the sympathetic nervous system (fight-or-flight response) and withdraws the parasympathetic nervous system (rest and digest). The accelerated heart rate, increased blood pressure, body stiffness, mental alertness, and hormonal changes within the body are prompting us to face a perceived dangerous situation. (There's more on the topic and effects of stress in Chapter 2.4).

In TCM terms, headaches can be a result of "over-ascending" Qi in anxious situations, meaning that too much energy is rushing upward to the head. When sudden gushes of Qi disrupt one's normal balanced order, discomfort or illness will result.

FUNCTIONS OF QI

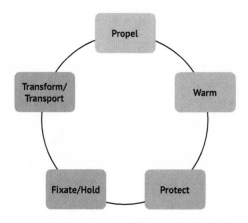

The functions of Qi

In addition to defining the directions of Qi, the Chinese have established five cardinal functions of Qi, as shown in the diagram and defined next: propel, warm, protect, fixate/hold, transform/transport.

- **Propel:** Qi stimulates and maintains the physiological functions of organs by propelling substances, blood, fluids, and liquids in the body. Think of it like filling a balloon: Air must be *pushed in* to fill (nourish) the balloon. Weak Qi will hinder the balloon's ability to expand. Thus, we say that a weakness of Qi can lead to deficiencies within the body. Qi also diminishes as one ages, expressed through the loss of appetite, decreased postural awareness, and muscle atrophy.

- **Warm:** Qi can produce heat and regulate body temperature for normal functions. There is an optimal temperature for the synthesis of life within the body. Healthy Qi sustains this environment. Therefore, unhealthy Qi would mean no warmth. That is why when someone lacks Qi, they typically have cold hands and feet and are cold averse.

- **Protect:** Healthy Qi can also form a barrier to protect humans from illness. With adequate amounts of healthy Qi, pathogens will have no way to invade the body. Unusual weather conditions (such as suddenly turning cold or hotter than usual) can sometimes favor what could be considered "unhealthy Qi," or sickness. When the unhealthy Qi is stronger than the healthy Qi in the body, we are more susceptible to sickness. More on weather later.

- **Fixate/Hold:** Imagine Qi as an invisible shopping bag that carries all sorts of things our body needs or produces. It provides a force that constrains and controls the liquid substances in our body, such as blood, body fluids, semen, menstrual blood, and others. Qi also stabilizes blood so that it flows inside the vessels instead of outside. It fixates body fluids to prevent runny noses and excessive sweating, which are symptoms of weak Qi fixation. Some people may see manifestations such as unusual sweating, drooling, diarrhea, and premature ejaculation.

- **Transport/Transform:** Qi is responsible for transforming the substances we take in (food, air) into blood or body fluids—all of which are vital essences of life.

QI: THE INTERCONNECTED WHOLE

As we've mentioned before, modern Western medicine focuses on the physical structures and functions of human bodies, whereas ancient TCM adopts a more philosophical approach, with concepts or abstractions that we are meant to interpret. Nowhere is that difference more evident than in this discussion about Qi.

Qi gives everything energy and life. Although the word Qi is usually translated into English as "energy," there are multiple facets to this powerful philosophical yet practical concept. TCM looks at the human body, nature, and the universe as interconnected systems linked by different kinds of Qi.

The implication that follows is that Qi is not just about living in harmony with our bodies but rather living in harmony with the world. It is this idea of connectedness that set the tone thousands of years ago for a natural way of living and natural therapeutic methods.

Blood: Nourishment of the Body

The first day back for the preseason, elite athletes will report to the sports medicine department for a comprehensive assessment. As part of the assessment, blood samples will be collected to assess the athletes' condition and overall health. Blood analysis is then carried out periodically throughout the season for purposes such as testing for drugs, evaluating lactate levels, and monitoring health.

Understanding the components and functions of blood is an integral part of Western medicine. Blood contains plasma, red blood cells, white blood cells, and platelets. It transports nutrients, delivers oxygen to the working muscles, removes metabolic waste, and regulates temperature.

The TCM understanding of blood is simpler and broader: Yes, blood is the red fluid inside the blood vessels that delivers nutrients to the body, but conceptually the term can be used to mean anything that brings nourishment to the body. Therefore, blood is vital to the mind and consciousness as well as physical functions.

FUNCTIONS OF BLOOD

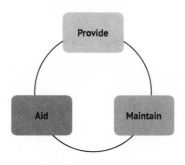

The functions of blood

TCM defines three important functions of blood, as shown in the previous figure and described next:

- **Provide:** Blood nourishes our organs and tissues for optimal
  function. The color tone of our skin and the condition of our
  nails, hair, muscles, and bones are the manifestations of how
  well our blood is nourishing our body to be strong and healthy.
  When blood circulation is poor (due to lack of sleep and exercise
  or cold weather, for example) and the blood is unable to properly
  nourish our body, we suffer from hair loss, fragile nails, bruises,
  rashes, or itches on the skin.

- **Maintain:** Blood maintains healthy sensations and body movements. The Chinese believed that injuries happen due to poor
  blood circulation. Poor blood circulation affects the nourishment of the body and thus can interrupt our sensory functions.
  Dizziness, ringing in the ear, and weak muscles are all examples
  of poor blood flow.

- **Aid:** Blood nourishes the mind, allowing us to enjoy good spir-
  its and swift reaction times. Sleep deprivation and unhealthy
  diets can reduce the body's ability to produce healthy blood and

eventually affect the nourishment of our mind, which can lead to outcomes such as poor memory, disrupted sleeping cycles, shortened attention spans, and even worse side effects in the long run.

QI AND BLOOD TO DESCRIBE CIRCULATION

Both Qi and blood can be used to describe circulation in isolation or combined. On the internet or in writing, you might see people referring to Qi and blood as "Qi-blood." Since there isn't a universal standard on the usage of these words, just be aware that these terms are referring to the same concept. That is, Qi can be evaluated on its own, blood can be evaluated on its own, and Qi and blood together can give us a fuller picture of the overall circulation. Ideally, the flow of Qi and blood will be well circulated without obstruction but not overstimulated, as it might lead to problems with balance in the body.

Activity: Evaluating Your Own Qi and Blood

As you can see, the proper movement of Qi and blood through the body is critical to health and performance. What about you? Are you aware of the health of your Qi and blood?

Here is a simple activity to check for balanced Qi and blood. Set the timer on your phone to five minutes and then switch it to airplane mode (with Wi-Fi off) so there won't be any distractions. During these five minutes, reflect on your health and performance over the past week.

After that, circle as many qualities in the following table as describe your recent experience.

HEALTH AND PERFORMANCE THE PAST WEEK

Category One

Motivated / Driven	Energetic / Good stamina
Curious / Imaginative	Peaceful
Happy / Joyful	Productive
Normal body temperature	Little to no pain
Smooth skin	Comfortable bowel movement

Category Two

Fatigue	Pain
Insomnia	Anxiety / Fear
Laziness / Procrastination	Stress / Tension
Sluggish bowel movements	Acne
Cold hands and feet	Prone to bruises

Where did you put the most circles? Category One or Two?

It probably didn't take you long to figure out Category One contains indicators of harmonious Qi and blood. As an athlete, who wouldn't want to be motivated, driven, and productive and have good stamina (all qualities of balanced Qi and blood)? Turns out, a lot of these qualities are influenced by your lifestyle choices, such as diet, movement, rest, and emotional management.

The outcomes of our lifestyle choices are actually quite intuitive in many cases. For example, imagine that you have a 10k race coming up this weekend. In preparation for optimal performance, you need balanced Qi, which includes good strength, stamina, motivation, and other qualities listed in Category One. You probably won't get a double cheeseburger with fries and a Coke before the race, as you instinctively know oily foods are not conducive to improved performance. Conversely, you probably will avoid going into the race on an empty stomach because there will be nothing to fuel your performance. Before the race, you may turn to music to either pump you up or calm your nerves, because you know from experience that you need to be motivated to perform at your best, but if you are overly stimulated, you will burn all your energy within the first few kilometers. The night before the race, you probably will look for a high-quality night of sleep. Not too much more than your usual duration because that will make you drowsy, but definitely not much less than your usual because intuitively you know that does not maximize your chances of success.

Again, Qi and blood are used to describe the overall functions of your body. Here is a challenge: The next time you order a meal at the restaurant or prepare your own, think about how what you eat might contribute to the qualities described in Category One. If you think what you are eating will maintain the health of your Qi and blood, make a special note of it. This will serve as your baseline, and your understanding of beneficial foods will most definitely change after reading this book.

If you are exhibiting more qualities from Category One, this signifies that you are relatively balanced. If you have more circles in Category Two, know that it is not the end of the world! Either way, you are on the right path, as this book will help you understand the underlying reasons behind different imbalances.

THE LANGUAGE OF BALANCE AND HARMONY (YIN-YANG AND FIVE PHASES)

The core belief of classical Chinese philosophy is that we humans should try to live in balance and harmony. That includes maintaining not just an *internal* dynamic balance within our bodies (homeostasis) but also an *external* balance, adjusting our lifestyles to stay in harmony with the natural world. The two TCM concepts covered in this chapter, Yin-Yang and the five phases, provide ideas and terms that we can use to describe what it takes to achieve balance and harmony both internally and externally.

Yin-Yang: The Balancing of Opposite Forces

 Terms in TCM are often expressed in pairs: Qi is usually paired with blood, Yin is paired with Yang, Zang is paired with Fu, just to name a few. Pairing might be a difficult concept to comprehend, especially for those of us who have been taught to think of everything in isolation. So why did the Chinese pair concepts together?

To help answer this question, think of the following idea: summer/ winter, day/night, happy/sad, tall/short, fast/slow, resilient/fragile, entertaining/boring. See the connections? Each of these represents opposite yet dependent forces that help us define the world we live in. Without one, the other wouldn't make sense. How could we define *happy* if we didn't know what *sad* meant? It is this concept of opposing forces in relation to each other that is critical to harmony and balance.

Many people in the West are familiar with Yin and Yang because of the ubiquitous Tai Chi sign, seen at the beginning of this chapter. But context and origin are important when it comes to understanding Yin and Yang.

HISTORICAL CONTEXT OF YIN AND YANG

In the historical text *Shuowen Jiezi*, a dictionary written during the Han dynasty (around 206 BC to 220 AD), Yin and Yang were a geographical reference used to describe directions.

China's latitude is slightly higher than the Tropic of Cancer (the farthest northern latitude at which the sun can appear directly overhead). The sun would shine on the southern side of the mountains in the Central Plain. The shady side of the mountains was referred to as Yin; the opposite sunny side was Yang. Ancient Chinese cities were named according to which side of the mountain they resided on (such as Luoyang and Nanyang).

However, just because one side is sunny and the other shady does not mean that one is superior to the other. Without the sunlight, there is no shade; without Yin, there is no Yang. The two forces are contradictory yet complementary. They are inseparable.

This interconnected nature of Yin and Yang is represented in the Tai Chi symbol, where the swirls represent two metaphorical fish: The white swirl represents the Yang fish, and the black swirl represents the Yin fish. When combined in balance, they create harmony and a complete circle of Yin and Yang. You may notice that there is a dot of the opposite color inside each swirl. This is because Yin and Yang are more than just an opposite of the other; they are also rooted in each other and can transform into the opposite element when conditions are met.

By understanding the origin, we now have a better impression of the characteristics and natures of Yin and Yang.

- Yin, the shady side of rivers and mountains, can be characterized as calm, downward, dim, feminine, and gentle and expressed by the dark, cold, water, winter, flats in music, humid weather, and valleys.

- Yang, the sunny side of rivers and mountains, can be characterized as an energetic vibe, upward, bright, masculine, and powerful and expressed by the light, hot, fire, summer, sharps in music, dry weather, and mountains.

The key idea is that Yin and Yang represent an inseparable pair, each keeping the other in balance. And it is that balance of opposites that you should keep in mind when making decisions about your own lifestyle and fitness routines.

Five Phases: Movement and Transition in Nature

Like Yin-Yang, the theory of five phases (*Wŭ-Xíng* in Chinese) is one of the main philosophical theories of medical practice in ancient China that has survived to present day. (It is sometimes referred to as the five elements. See the "'Elements' vs. 'Phases'" sidebar.) The five phases are wood, fire, earth, metal, and water, and each has its own characteristics.

A full description of the phases and their characteristics is beyond the scope of this book, but here are some examples of how ancient scholars described them:

- Wood can be bent and straightened.
- Fire flares upward.
- Earth permits sowing, growing, and reaping.
- Metal can be molded and hardened.
- Water moistens downward.

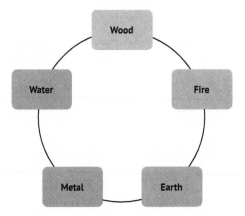

Though the five phases can be represented in different ways, the components are always arranged in a particular order (fire comes after wood, earth comes after fire, and so on) to represent the idea that nature cycles through stages of transition.

The phases are applied to make sense of different phenomena occurring around us (remember the Chinese made sense of the world through connections). Unlike in TV shows and other products of pop culture (such as *Avatar: The Last Airbender*, *Naruto*, and *Pokémon*), where the phases are sometimes interpreted as supernatural elements with opposing or strengthening effects, TCM sees these five materials as dynamic phases of nature's law. These phases are more than just substances that show certain qualities and characteristics. They represent different properties, phases, and relationships observed in nature.

"Elements" vs. "Phases"

As with Yin-Yang, a little historical context can help us understand how the five phases evolved and what they represent. According to ancient literature, *Wŭ-Xíng* was meant to be a short form of *Wŭ* (five) *Xíng* (moving) *Xīn* (stars). Originally, the "five moving stars" were named after planets, which denoted movement and activity. As time when on, scholars redefined *Wŭ-Xíng* as an abstract concept represented by basic materials (wood, fire, earth, metal, water).

The word *elements* (as in "five elements") was then applied to describe these basic materials. The problem with using the word *elements*, however, is that an ordinary person would not associate the concept of an element with movement and activity, which was the original intent of *Wŭ-Xíng*. Therefore, instead of using the term "five elements," scholars have called for the use of either "five phases" (which implies activity) or just *Wŭ-Xíng* itself. Our book uses "five phases" rather than "five elements" to emphasize the ever-changing nature of the phases.

Applying Yin-Yang and Five Phases to Performance Enhancement

As you'll see in Part 2, the most obvious application of the Yin-Yang and five phases concepts involves making decisions about your lifestyle and training to maintain balance and order. Here are some examples.

YIN-YANG AND BALANCE IN TRAINING

From a micro perspective, vigorous exercises during a training session would be considered Yang, whereas the warm-up and the cooldown are Yin. Based on the Yin-Yang philosophy, the warm-up and recovery parts of the workout are of equal importance to any exercises or activities. If you go straight to training by ignoring the warm-up and end a session without a cooldown, you are acutely challenging the balance of your body and exposing yourself to a greater risk of injury.

If we take a macro perspective and look at training as a whole, the training session would be Yang (energy/power) and the recovery periods in between sessions would be Yin (calmness). Therefore, intense training sessions must be paired with quality recovery periods. If you do not allow time for your body to recover in between strenuous training sessions, the body will never perform at an optimal level.

The subtitle of our book indicates the grand objective of athletic performance enhancement. Generally, books that pertain to the topic of strength and conditioning would include a focus on training methodologies that get an athlete bigger, faster, and stronger: "What can you do to build strength, power, and endurance?"

Our book began by posing a seemingly opposite question: "How can you *recover* better?" We must pay as much attention to the recovery—the ability to maintain dynamic balance—as we do to the actual training. Without adequate recovery, performance enhancement is just an afterthought.

Understanding the concept of Yin and Yang and its relationship with nature is vital for us to better understand ourselves. The truth is, workout routines, training strategies, dietary plans, and emotions should not be the same year-round. Changes and adaptations should be made according to the subtle yet dynamic change in Yin-Yang for us to feel better, live better, and perform better.

If you haven't already, incorporate recovery strategies into your daily routine; that can be things such as stretching, massage, foam rolling, mobility workouts, breathing, and meditation. Take note of what type of recovery strategies you prefer.

ESTABLISHING HARMONY WITH THE SEASONS: YIN-YANG AND FIVE PHASES

In the Introduction, we established the need to maintain dynamic balance internally—the range of slightly changing equilibrium where one achieves optimal athletic performance. To achieve that state of internal equilibrium, many high-performing athletes are already paying a great deal of attention to their lifestyle choices. Many are following an optimal diet or optimal sleeping schedule, while others might be reading up on other disciplines that can improve different aspects of their health and well-being.

But as you can now see, our external environment should also influence the lifestyle that we live. We must live in harmony with the world. Not only are we designed to do so, but harmonious living externally, with nature and the world, can ultimately influence the body internally. The Chinese believe there are five seasons: spring, summer, late summer, autumn, and winter.

For example, as shown in the following figure, summer to autumn, as the hottest time of year, is the "Yang of Yang," the peak expression of the energetic (hot) season. Autumn to winter is the "Yin of Yang," a time where temperatures start to drop and heat and energy in nature are diminishing, which brings us cool and calm (serene) weather. Animals begin to hibernate, and plants start withering to conserve energy for the transformation. The transition from winter to spring, the "Yin of Yin," is the low-energy ebb of the low-energy season and is usually the coldest time of the year. Most organisms (other than humans) take a break and rest in their dens, waiting for nature's recovery. Spring to summer is the "Yang of Yin": Life grows vividly as the cold gradually makes its way out of this stage. Ice melts, plants bud out, bugs come out of the soil, and animals begin mating. During this transition, "Yang" regains its dominancy in the universe. Transition periods between seasons, or anytime when nature changes from Yin to Yang (or vice versa), are important because they prepare the body for what's to come.

SEASON CHANGES

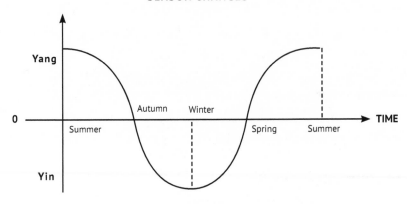

The five seasons, Yin, and Yang

Just as each season has its own Yin or Yang characteristics, it is also associated with one of the five phases.

- Wood represents spring because spring is a season of growth. In spring, plants are gaining energy from their surroundings to bloom later in the summer.

- Summer is a time of maximum activity or greatest Yang, so it is represented by fire.

- Late summer corresponds to the earth phase as the season of nourishment.

- Autumn is a season of reaping and harvest, bleak and solemn, when energy is stored. This is associated with metal, focusing on precision and organization as one plans ahead for winter.

- Winter, relating to water, is the season of rest. Energy is conserved beneath the soil, waiting until spring comes again.

These concepts might sound abstract to you now, but we will refer to the Yin-Yang and five phases in later chapters as we ask you to examine whether your lifestyle is matching the current phase of the season that you are in. As we'll discuss, one of the causes for imbalance—and seemingly inexplicable challenges in achieving performance or lifestyle goals—is that we are not eating and living in accordance with the current season. In other words, being in sync with the seasons (and hence phases) is key to maintaining balance and harmony with nature; being out of sync can lead to problems that interfere with your athletic performance. We'll also use the characteristics of the five phases to explain how you can adjust your activities or design a training schedule that better suits whichever phase you are in.

To help you start thinking about how to get in harmony with nature, take a minute (or ten!) to look at the world around you. What is the current season as you read this book? What does the natural world look and feel like where you are currently?

At the time we are writing this chapter, for example, it is getting warm and humid here in Hong Kong because it is spring. The earth is coming alive again. Grasses and trees are turning green and growing new shoots. New flowers are opening, and the air is filled with the sweet scent of blossoms and the sounds of birds singing. Many people are out hiking to enjoy stunning views of nature.

The seasonal phase where you are probably does not match our description. It could be a different season, or you could live in an area where the signs of the seasons are quite different from what we see in Hong Kong.

THE BODY IS NOT A MACHINE (ZANG-FU AND MERIDIANS)

In Western medicine, the body is often viewed as a complicated machine with a number of isolated and independent parts. Any illness or sickness means that some part of the machine is malfunctioning. To fix the machine, the physician just needs to fix the affected parts. And as long as you can fix the affected parts, the problem can be solved—or so the accepted thinking goes.

Take high blood pressure, for example. Instead of identifying the root cause of the problem, patients are commonly prescribed beta blockers that suppress the communication between the brain and the body. This approach does include risks, such as some common side effects and the risk of being dependent on the medication. But then, risks in the medical field are deemed tolerable as long as the sickness is healed.

Make no mistake, Western medicine has provided life-changing tools to fix acute problems such as accidental injuries and life-threatening diseases. However, it often overlooks the need to identify and address the root cause of the problem. In recent years, there have been calls for a form of medicine that considers the whole person in the quest for optimal health and wellness. That is, instead of viewing body parts as separate and independent components, they should be viewed as interdependent and considered as part of a comprehensive medical plan.

That is exactly the approach taken in TCM. The Chinese have long viewed the body as a whole with interdependent parts. The connection between organs is expressed through the two concepts we will discuss in this chapter: Zang-Fu organs and meridians. Zang-Fu categorizes the organs according to the functions they perform in the body. Meridians are paths that transport the Qi and blood of the body, and they connect the Zang-Fu organs and the rest of the body.

Zang-Fu Theory

The Zang-Fu theory is how TCM treats the internal organs of the human body. *Zang* translates as "to hide" or "to store," and *Fu* means "a repository or warehouse." However, unlike the Western view of human bodies, Zang-Fu theory does not treat an organ as a fixed anatomical structure (stomach, liver, heart, etc.). The need to systematically describe bodily functions was more important to ancient TCM physicians than giving names to individual structures (more on this later). Therefore, Zang-Fu can be better understood as functions that have loose anatomical associations.

Here again, we run into a key difference between Western medicine and TCM. The West takes a microscopic approach and views organs as separate parts. These individual organs can be examined and studied using modern technology. Zang-Fu and more broadly TCM are based on the concept of holism. Taking a macroscopic approach, TCM views the human body as a dynamic system that is constantly changing, adapting, and interacting with the external environment and internal emotions. The organs cannot be separated from other forces that are influencing how the body functions as a whole. By observing and interpreting the manifestation of Zang-Fu, we can better understand what is happening inside us.

Zang-Fu is divided into three categories: Zang, Fu, and extraordinary organs. The following table shows an overview of the Zang and Fu aspects.

ZANG AND FU SUMMARY

	Zang	Fu
Structures or associated organs	Commonly referred to as the five organs: • Liver • Heart & Pericardium • Spleen • Lungs • Kidneys	• Gallbladder • Stomach • Small intestine • Large intestine • Urinary bladder • The triple burner (this has no corresponding meaning in Western medicine—see sidebar)
Nature	Yin (calm, downward)	Yang (energetic, upward)
Functions	Manufacture and store the vital substances (Qi, Blood, and certain essences).	They transform our food and drink into essences to nourish the Zang and other parts of the body. Some of these essences are later stored in the Zang organs. Fu organs do not store. A healthy Fu organ should be in a constant cycle of being filled and emptied.
The Yellow Emperor's Classic of Medicine*	The five Zang organs are solid, installing but not discharging. They can be full of essential Qi instead of containing foodstuffs.	The six Fu organs are hollow, discharging but not installing. They can be full of foodstuff instead of storing essential Qi.
Interpretation and application	One should adopt a lifestyle that protects the five organs. One should avoid overusing the Zang such as staying up all night, excessive drinking, and excessive eating.	Fu should have a dynamic recurring cycle of being filled and being emptied. If the Fu is not emptied in time, it becomes congested and stuck. However, if the Fu is being emptied too fast and cannot get filled, one might experience symptoms such as diarrhea.

*The Yellow Emperor's Classic of Medicine, or Huangdi Neijing, is an ancient Chinese medicine text that has been viewed as one of the fundamental TCM doctrines.

What Is the Triple Burner?

The TCM concept of the triple burner (or *sān jiāo* in Chinese) has no correlation in Western medicine at this time. The triple burner is more a function of the human body than a specific organ. *Triple* corresponds roughly to the three parts of the human torso (above the diaphragm, between the diaphragm and navel, and below the navel). *Burner* (or sometimes *energizer*) refers to the function of allowing the free flow of Qi in the body.

EXTRAORDINARY FU

The third category is known as the extraordinary Fu. This group of organs shares the characteristics of Zang and Fu and refers to the brain, marrow, bone, blood vessels, gallbladder, and uterus. Like Zang, they also store vital substances, and like Fu, they are hollowed but can be closed or concealed. They do not contact with foodstuffs directly.

Unlike the pairing of Zang and Fu, extraordinary organs do not share a Yin and Yang relationship. They are independent, hence the name "extraordinary."

THE ZANG ORGANS AND PERFORMANCE

Throughout the rest of this book, we will talk mostly about the Zang organs, how they exhibit signs of our health and well-being (or lack thereof), and how this relates to identifying and resolving issues with athletic performance. We will not talk much about the Fu organs, not because they are inferior to the Zang organs but because Fu organs share similar physiological functions: digestion, absorption, and excretion of food and fluids. While these are important functions for the body, looking at individual Fu organs does not help us as much in improving fitness and performance.

The following table will help you understand how the TCM view of the five organs compares to the Western view. As you can see, the functions are not strictly physiological.

ZANG ORGANS OVERVIEW

Zang	Functions as defined in TCM	How imbalances can affect athletic performance
Liver	• Modulates the flow of Qi and stores blood • Connects the tendons and manifests in our nails and eyes • Regulates emotions • Assists the function of the spleen and stomach	• Recurrent joint pain / discomfort • Muscle stiffness • Bad eyesight
Heart	• Governs the blood and the vessels • House to the Mind • Manifests in the tongue	• Impaired stamina / endurance • Dizziness • Prone to mental distractions
Heart (Pericardium)	• Considered to be part of the heart as well, so shares the same features with the heart	
Spleen	• Aids the stomach in the digestion of food • Transforms nutrients from food and liquids to energy to nourish different parts of the body • Governs muscle growth • Restrains blood to flow in the vessels (prevents bleeding and bruising)	• Poor digestion • Trouble building muscle mass • Weak muscles • Prone to unexplained bruises
Lungs	• Control Qi and respiration • Regulate water ways such as the circulation of body fluids • Sending inhaled air to the spleen so that they (air + food in the spleen) can be transformed into energy	• Low stamina • Poor immune system
Kidney	• Stores nutrients and modulates our body fluids • Governs growth and reproduction • Dictates the deepness of breath—the origin of energies (inherited from our parents) of the entire body	• Bone and joint discomfort • Lower back soreness • Prone to dizziness

The Meridian System

Through centuries of medical practice and observation, the ancient physicians discovered continuous inner body channels or pathways through which life energy (Qi) is circulated. These pathways are called meridians. They cannot be observed by the naked eye; they do not appear as physical structures.

Meridians and Acupuncture

Meridians are extensively studied by acupuncturists, because the job of acupuncturists is to adjust the flow of Qi by inserting needles along the meridian pathways. The places where needles are inserted are often called acupuncture points.

Meridians have physiological functions that are critical to one's well-being. They transport Qi and blood to different parts of the body. Visceral organs are connected to the superficial and deep tissues via the meridians. The meridians also reflect pathological changes of the visceral organs. With such vital functions, it is important for athletes to maintain smooth energy flow and avoid stagnation.

When we use the term *chan*, we are usually referring to the twelve regular meridians of the body. The Qi and blood flow in these are the strongest. These meridians also connect internal organs with the torso and external limbs. The 12 Meridians are illustrated in the following figures and can be categorized according to their routes as follows:

- Three Yang meridians in the arms
    - » Large Intestine Meridian
    - » Triple Burner Meridian
    - » Small Intestine Meridian

- Three Yin meridians in the arms
  - » Lung Meridian
  - » Pericardium Meridian
  - » Heart Meridian
- Three Yang meridians in the legs
  - » Stomach Meridian
  - » Bladder Meridian
  - » Gallbladder Meridian
- Three Yin meridians in the legs
  - » Spleen Meridian
  - » Liver Meridian
  - » Kidney Meridian

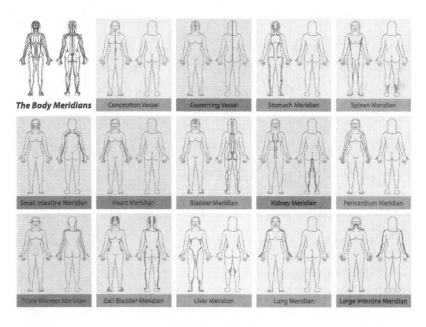

The Body Meridians

Yin and Yang meridians were classified from the sunlight that they would receive. That is, there was a time when human ancestors were on all fours. In this orientation, the back side would face the sky and receive more sunlight (a Yang characteristic). The front side of the body, facing downward, received less sunlight (a Yin characteristic).

The hand and feet Yin and Yang meridians are segments of meridians that interconnect to form a longer pathway. This pathway connects our body from head to toe, from inside to the outside. Qi, blood, and other materials that flow in these meridians are then transported to nourish our body.

The meridian system is like a traffic network of highways, roads, and streets that links different cities. The highways (meridians) and the cities (Zang-Fu) make up the entire body map. There are other, smaller branches, called collaterals, that can be thought of as the roads and streets. It is through this traffic network that life energy (Qi) is transported.

Many factors can affect the overall efficiency of the traffic network. Poor weather like rainy days or snow days may slow down traffic flow. Roads that are poorly maintained (such as an unhealthy lifestyle) will make drivers slow down. Traffic accidents (sports injuries), and even those dreaded slow drivers (Qi and blood stagnation), will also cause traffic congestion.

On the flip side, reckless drivers (caffeine, drugs, too hyped up) going over the speed limit (excessive flow of Qi and blood) are not helping the system either. Even though it may seem as though they get to the destination ahead of schedule, the cities may not be able to accommodate them (excessive Qi and blood rushing to the head can cause headaches and fever).

DIRECTION OF FLOW

It's also helpful to know the general flow direction of meridian types, as that has a profound implication in TCM strategies to overcome imbalances. A summary of the meridians and their energy flow is shown in the following table. An in-depth discussion of their impact on TCM treatments is beyond the scope of this book, but you'll find a summary of several key points in Appendix B regarding the significance in TCM treatments.

MERIDIAN TYPES AND DIRECTION OF ENERGY FLOW

Meridian Type	Direction of Flow
Yin meridians of the arms	Chest to arms
Yang meridians of the arms	Arms to head
Yang meridians of the leg	Head to foot
Yin meridians of the leg	Foot to chest

The Body as a Whole

As we learned in this chapter, the relationship between Zang-Fu and meridians is analogous to the transportation system between cities. Just like how a highway could not exist without destinations, the meridians cannot exist without Zang-Fu.

Understanding the interplay between different Zang-Fu organs and meridians is critical to understanding how TCM views the interconnected body as a whole. While each Zang-Fu organ has a unique function, the overarching principle is that all of them are closely related to each other for optimal health and performance. Deficiencies in one location will result in a cascade of deficiencies elsewhere.

Take some time now to reflect on your athletic journey. Which Zang-Fu imbalances have you experienced in your athletic career?

THE SEARCH FOR SMOOTH AND ELEGANT MOVEMENTS (MUSCLES AND FASCIA)

The study of human anatomy can be dated back thousands of years. Just as we've seen in the previous chapters, in the West, human musculature has been treated as a collection of individual components. Anatomy textbooks would outline how each skeletal muscle functions through understanding how it attaches to bones, other tissues, or muscles. Health and fitness professionals were taught that each muscle had specific actions. (For example, the rectus femoris, one of the four quadriceps muscles, attaches from the pelvis to below the knee joint. Therefore, it flexes the hip and extends the knee.)

In light of this, many gyms are filled with big machines to work specific muscle groups. If you want to train your rectus femoris, you would jump on the machine that requires knee-extension or hip-flexion movement.

Over time, gym enthusiasts develop their routine according to these individual muscle groups around a particular body area. The following table is a suggested five-day split in an article titled "What Is the Best 5-Day Workout Split?" from the popular website bodybuilding.com.

Example 5-Day Workout

Monday	Universal Chest Day / Abs
Tuesday	Back / Abs
Wednesday	Legs
Thursday	Rest
Friday	Chest /Abs
Saturday	Back / Abs
Sunday	Shoulders and Arms / Abs

The routine is based on a traditional understanding of anatomy—that each muscle, when looked at in isolation, is a unique combination of three types of actions: concentric (shortening), eccentric (lengthening), and isometric (maintaining current length). To many people, it makes perfect sense that muscles have to be targeted specifically. Muscles are understood through a model of opposites known as agonist-antagonist pairs. That is, the main muscle (agonist) contracts concentrically to produce a movement as the opposite muscle (antagonist) lengthens.

But how does this view compare with real life? Let's go back to Andy's story about his high school days when he signed up for training sessions to become a better soccer player, which we talked about in the Introduction. Due credit to the trainer, because he did conduct an often overlooked yet critical step of the assessment process: a needs analysis. The goal of this analysis is to identify the physical demands of a sport and subsequently identify which physical qualities or movements are most important for the athlete to perform well in their sport. As Andy talked about his lofty ambitions of playing college soccer, the trainer gave him a quick rundown on his needs. And the guidance went something like this:

"Imagine kicking a ball with your right (or left) leg. Right at the moment of impact, as you are swinging your leg from back to front, you are flexing the hips. Meanwhile, the knee of the kicking leg also is moving into extension for maximal power. Combining the two moves, the plan is to strengthen the muscles that produce hip flexion and knee extension. That way, you can kick the ball farther and outperform others."

That summer, Andy did a lot of leg raises on the hanging leg-raise machine, where he would place both forearms on the pads and raise his legs upward to a point that is parallel to the ground. For knee extensions, he would jump into the knee-extension machine. He would sit in the chair, bend his knees, and set up the pad so that it sat on top of his shoelaces. Then he would extend his knee to move against the resistance of the pad.

After weeks of dedicated training, Andy returned to the United States for the start of the school year. One afternoon, while shopping for school supplies, he visited some clothing stores to ensure that he looked fresh returning to school. To his surprise, he had trouble buying clothes, especially pants. His upper body fit comfortably into a size small shirt. But while his waist size was about 27 inches, he could not fit into any jeans or pants. The jeans were super tight, and in those days, it was embarrassing to wear tightly fitted jeans at his school. So in the end he had to buy jeans that were 30 inches.

Turns out, his muscle-focused training had worked, in a way. His thighs were massive in relation to his waist.

But more important, did that lead to better performance?

Andy says he can tell you for sure that he did not kick the ball farther even with bigger thighs, even if he kicked it as hard as he could. If anything, he found that muscle size and power are not positively related after a certain point. That is, having adequate leg muscles to support different movements is important, but too much does not necessarily translate to stronger performance.

Here is the bottom line: Twenty years ago, it was natural for a trainer to think about muscles in isolation when it came to performance enhancement. In fact, the prevailing emphasis of training has always been on muscle training and cardiovascular conditioning. But now, trainers who are applying only isolated muscle training are sorely missing out on the advances in health science.

An emerging topic in health science, certainly within exercise science, is giving us another perspective on human anatomy and muscular function. New findings are pointing to the fact that a bigger network is at the heart of human movement and function. Namely, the fascial network.

How Do We Produce Movement?

The contractile component of tissues—so called because it produces the tension and contractions that allow us to move—has long been the focus of exercise science textbooks. That is, a muscle contracts when its component filaments slide against each other.

As you may know, however, there is also a noncontractile component of tissues, which gives a muscle or other tissue its shape or form. These include ligaments, joint capsules, and fascia.

A growing understanding of that last noncontractile tissue, fascia, is revolutionizing the way we look at health, and the way we train. Fascia, which is the Latin word for "band" and is pronounced "fah-sha," can be thought of as a spiderweb that permeates throughout the entire body. It is a type of connective tissue that forms sheets or bands beneath the skin to attach, stabilize, enclose, and separate muscles and other internal organs. Without fascia holding us together, we would be nothing but a mess of jelly.

Different types of fasciae can be found throughout the body. For the purposes of this book, the type of fascia we want to concentrate on is the myofascia. *Myo* is from the Greek word for "muscle," so myofascia describes the fascia that wraps around the muscles.

The traditional notion that fascia in the human body mainly functioned only to "hold things together" is a natural conclusion, because fascia creates the compartments and shapes of the different muscles that we see. Nonetheless, the understanding of fascia has evolved. Research now tells us that our central nervous system receives a great amount of sensory input from myofascial tissues. Within the layer of myofascial tissues are different sensory nerve endings (mechanoreceptors) that are able to detect pressure and length changes. These sensory nerve endings have been found within muscles (intramuscular) and outside the muscles (extramuscular), such as in the fascial tissues, beneath the skin.

While fascia allows muscles to glide and move, it also plays a role in four other important biological functions that we want to mention because these concepts come up frequently when talking about the mechanisms of TCM practices:

1. **Proprioception:** Even if you close your eyes, you still know where your left hand or right foot or hip or elbow is positioned and are aware of their movements, though you cannot see them. The body's awareness of itself in space is called proprioception.

2. **Nociception:** Is any part of your body in pain? The way you know this is nociception.

3. **Exteroception:** Wherever and whenever you're reading this book, you probably know what the environment outside of your body is like—the air temperature, humidity, sounds, smells, and so on. That awareness of the external environment is exteroception.

4. **Interoception:** How is your body feeling right now? The sense of the body's internal state is interoception.

Fascial Properties

Renowned fascia researchers Robert Schleip, PhD, and Jan Wilke, PhD, listed several important insights about fascia in the updated edition of their comprehensive book *Fascia in Sport and Movement.*

- Fascial tissues react to everyday strain as well as specific training.
- Fascial tissues will respond in a process of constant repair and remodeling if stimulated.
- Fascial tissues are capable of storing and releasing kinetic energy similar to an elastic spring.
- Force generation depends on the fascia's ability to lengthen before a contraction.

Since the fascial network surrounds and penetrates the entire human body, any local dysfunction or even poorly managed emotions can have an adverse effect on how the fascia functions, and therefore on the body as a whole. Instead of being smooth, elastic, and slippery, unhealthy fascia becomes sticky, rigid, or even clumpy.

Here's another way to think about it: The human body has long been thought of as a post-and-beam skyscraper—the bones are the main structure, and the soft tissues and muscles are the supporting walls. A major flaw with this approach is that the human body is not a rigid, lifeless structure; rather, it is a mobile and flexible living organism that adapts to the surrounding environment. Here is how Thomas Myers, a pioneer in the field of fascial movement and training, described the modern understanding of fascia in an interview on *HuffPost:* "Real fascia in real people is very fluid, very dynamic, and has these kinds of plastic . . . properties that allow us to change in ways that we haven't thought we could open and change."[1] As Myers pointed out, fascia is fluid and dynamic; it is elastic and flexible.

---

1   Norlyk Smith, E. 2014. "Creating Change: Tom Myers on Yoga, Fascia and Mind-Body Transformation." HuffPost.com. February 5, 2014. Retrieved December 26, 2020, from https://www.huffpost.com/entry/mind-body-_b_4387093.

Healthy Fascia

- Gummy
- Sticky
- Crinkled Up

- Smooth
- Slippery
- Flexible

Tensegrity = Tension + Integrity

To better understand healthy fascia, we first must understand the term *tensegrity*, which is a combination of *tension* and *integrity*. It refers to the dynamic tension that our bodies and muscles must maintain in order for us to function and move.

Tensegrity is based on an architectural concept created by renowned American architect and inventor Buckminster Fuller. But it can help us understand the relationship between fascia and human movement. The concept of tensegrity holds that different components of something (a building or body) are under constant pressure, and those components are arranged in such a way that they do not touch each other.

This concept is easier to understand with visual models, such as the example shown in the following figures that represent the human body. The rods (bones) are held together by elastic cords (muscle and fascia). The integrity of a structure (your body) is derived from the balance of the tension members (your muscles and fascia), not the compression struts (the bones). The tensegrity in this model is the ideal amount of tension and elasticity that allows it to maintain form but still move. In the same way, dynamic balance is your body's ability to maintain tensegrity as you move.

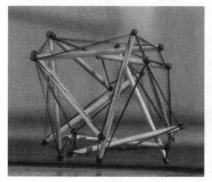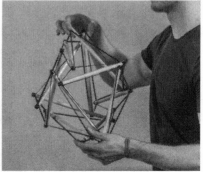

Example of tensegrity

We encourage you to purchase a tensegrity model (or make your own) because playing with these models helps you better understand how fascia and other internal structures respond when you move. Force applied to any single part of a tensegrity structure affects the whole form. Most important, you'll see that compression or decompression in one area can cause tension in another. Therefore, when we examine examples of imbalance—such as postural compensation, discomfort, and pain—using the principles of tensegrity, we look along the lines of tension in your body. The source of your discomfort may not be the part that appears squashed or stretched. It may even be a place that is seemingly unrelated. (We'll refer to the tensegrity model in Part 3 of this book when we discuss strategies such as movement, cupping, and Gua Sha.)

Healthy fascia is integral to movement, emotion, and overall health. Imbalance within the three-dimensional net of fascia would drastically hinder performance, as it would increase your risk of injury.

Fascial Training

Fascial meridians, or fascial lines, are line-like structures that permeate and surround the entire body. Take the superficial front line, for example. It connects the entire front side of the body, from the top of the feet to the skull, as one continuous myofascial line in two pieces:

toes to the pelvis, then pelvis to head. (See Appendix B for a full list of the meridians and their properties.)

These lines have a profound impact on the way health and fitness professionals approach training. When someone is kicking a ball, for example, power is generated not only from the hip flexors or knee extensors but also from the entire superficial front line. Imagine yourself as a soccer player wanting to get the ball fifty yards downfield, or an American football kicker who can win a game with a fifty-yard field goal. Before your foot hits the ball, what do you do? Your *forward* kicking movement must be preceded by a *backward* movement of your leg. And what happens as you swing your leg back? The entire front line is stretched and extended, and mechanical energy is stored (loaded) in the tendons and fascia as well as the muscles. Then, as you bring your leg forward, energy is released as soon as the front line is released (unloaded), very much like a stretched rubber band snapping back into its normal shape.

This load-unload sequence can be found in every efficient sporting movement and extends to all activities of daily living. Humans have been utilizing this mechanism for as long as we have existed. Think of jumping: You typically do a small dip (load) before you explode off the floor (unload). Think of throwing a heavy bag of trash into those big and tall dumpsters: You do some sort of winding up (load) with the bag before you let it fly into the dumpster (unload).

Now go back to the isolated training concept where a soccer player or football kicker focuses on training the muscles that bring the hip into flexion and knee into extension. Imagine if the player only kicks the ball using pure muscular power, no loading, no momentum of any sort. Do you think the ball can still travel fifty yards? In the same way, imagine that you are instructed to jump as high as possible while seated on a chair, or toss the heavy trash bag without any swinging movement. How do you think you will do? Better or worse than with the small dip for jumping or the swing of the bag?

Training the fascial lines as an interconnected whole through integrated total body movements better mimics the movements that are required for any sport, thereby leading to better ability to move. And this is why healthy fascia is critical for—and we'd go so far as to say a prerequisite to—optimal athletic performance.

Imagine you are assembling your own slingshot right now. You have a Y-shaped stick in front of you and need to attach the band that will provide the propulsion. You have three bands to choose from: (1) a rigid and sticky band made of taffy, (2) a flexible and smooth band made of rubber, and (3) a thin band that lacks any tension, like an overstretched piece of elastic. Common sense should tell you that the flexible and smooth rubber band—which has balanced tension and integrity—will give you the best results. It will stretch more and more easily than choices 1 or 3, thereby storing and producing greater power, and will rebound to its original shape. This principle holds true for your muscular and fascial network as well. A well-maintained fascial network, with the right tension and integrity, can unlock your movement capabilities, to produce those effortless, silky, elegant, yet powerful movements that the best athletes make.

In the case of Andy's soccer story, if he has strong thigh muscles but does not learn to use them as part of a load-unload sequence, he's just wasting energy. Looking back, Andy thinks it was foolish of him to think that he had to kick "as hard as I possibly could" for the ball to travel fifty yards. If you look at the best players in the World Cup, you will see that without much of a blunt effort, they can make the ball travel in the air for fifty yards from one side of the field to the other.

Finding Balance: Isolated Muscle vs. Total Body Movement

Knowing the importance of fascial training through integrated exercises, some health and fitness professionals have abandoned isolated muscular training. Inexplicably, fitness-related methodologies always seem to be taken to the extremes. There are times when isolated muscle training is applicable and relevant, such as during rehabilitation, or when the muscle is found to be significantly weak during the initial fitness assessment.

A major point that we want to continually demonstrate throughout this book is the idea of finding balance in virtually everything: understanding the Yin and the Yang of a concept and avoiding the trap of moving into an extreme, unless the situation demands it. That's why the balanced approach of TCM would not rule out the idea of isolated muscle training entirely.

Are Fascial Meridians and TCM Meridians the Same Thing?

In the previous chapters, we talked about how the TCM view has it that optimal health requires unobstructed flow of energy through the channels of meridians. Here, we've talked about how the fascial meridians are key to our ability to maintain tensegrity and are integral to our physical and emotional well-being. Since TCM has never proved the physical existence of meridians, could it be that the fascial meridians are the anatomical basis of TCM meridians?

Professor Yu Bai of Southern Medical University and colleagues provided some insight on this issue when they published a review in 2011 in the peer-reviewed journal *Evidence-Based Complementary and Alternative Medicine* to evaluate evidence suggesting that the fascial network could be the anatomical basis for acupoints and meridians. They evaluated studies that looked at the human body through computed tomography and magnetic resonance imaging, and also studies that examined the physiological role of fascia. After evaluating the available evidence, they wrote in the discussion section that "the anatomy of the fascial network in the human body is consistent with the traditional view of the meridian network pattern." They went on to call for more research in examining the relationship between the two.

continued

The short answer is that right now we don't know for sure. But the two concepts are both treated as useful ideas that help us view the body as an interconnected whole, not isolated parts. If you'd like to read more about fascia and meridians, we highly recommend the engaging and popular book *The Spark in the Machine*, by Daniel Keown.

Developing Elegance in Your Movements

In her article on connective tissues in the journal *Medical Hypotheses*, Helene Langevin, a medical doctor and professor at the University of Vermont, succinctly stated a theme we've incorporated in our book: that a more holistic approach to medicine, in which the body's interconnections and interactions are considered, is needed moving forward.

We hope that the discussion of tensegrity, fascia, muscles, and meridians in this chapter has given you a deeper understanding of why we can't treat our bodies like machines in which isolated parts can be fixed or improved. We are all living, breathing humans striving for elegant movements and good health.

What does this mean in practice? If you have been doing a lot of isolated muscle work, you don't necessarily have to stop everything you're used to doing. Rather, look for balance that works the whole system of muscles and fascia needed for your sport. Chapter 3.3 describes the Five Animal Movements routine that you can try at home (with more details in Chapter 4.6). Feel free to jump ahead to take a sneak peek, but to get the most out of this book, we recommend continuing to follow the sequence as prepared.

PIECING TOGETHER THE EAST AND THE WEST

Henan University researcher Jie-hua Wang pointed out in an article published in the *Chinese Journal of Integrative Medicine* that the core value of TCM is to *help humans maintain their ability to adapt to nature.* If the body is not able to continually cope with the vagaries of the outside environment, we will not be able to maintain our dynamic equilibrium, resulting in a number of health or fitness challenges.

The following table shows how the TCM concepts that we have covered in the previous chapters are related to each other and to nature. As you can see, the five phases are used to categorize and explain a wide array of phenomena, from the seasons and climate to the interactions between the internal organs, and even taste (we will learn more about the concept of taste in Chapter 2.3). Keep in mind that the five phases are always moving, interconnected and interdependent on each other. They cannot exist without the others.

UNDERSTANDING THE CONNECTIVITY OF NATURE

Nature			Phase	Human Body			
Season	Climate	Taste		Zang Organ	Fu Organ	Body Tissue	Emotion
Spring	Wind	Sour	Wood	Liver	Gallbladder	Tendon	Anger
Summer	Heat	Bitter	Fire	Heart	Small Intestine and Triple Burner*	Vessels	Joy
Late Summer	Damp	Sweet	Earth	Spleen	Stomach	Muscle	Worry and Pensive-ness
Autumn	Dryness	Spicy	Metal	Lung	Large Intes-tine	Skin	Grief
Winter	Cold	Salty	Water	Kidney	Urinary Bladder	Bone	Fear and Fright

*Triple burner is sometimes categorized as the fire phase in acupuncture theory, but it is also referred to as a lone organ—one that does not fit into any category.

In the rest of the book, we're going to show you how to integrate the concepts covered in the previous chapters—Qi, blood, Yin-Yang, five phases, Zang-Fu, meridians, and fascia—into your own thinking about how to establish and maintain optimal health and performance. As you'll see, one of the biggest benefits of using TCM concepts lies in identifying how imbalances occur and ways to correct them.

PART 2

SEEKING SOURCES OF IMBALANCE AND FATIGUE

UNDERSTANDING THE DEPLETED BODY

After reading Part 1, you should have an awareness of some key concepts associated with traditional Chinese medicine. TCM principles can add to your understanding of how to achieve optimal fitness and performance by helping you to identify potential causes of imbalance that you might not be aware of if you only pay attention to Western medicine and fitness practices. In this part, we lay out principles to identify and determine the root causes of imbalance.

To kick off this section of the book, we'd like you to take a few minutes to complete a quick questionnaire (Chapter 2.1) that will indicate which aspects of your body functions are in or out of harmony according to TCM principles. After that, we'll present a case study (Chapter 2.2) and use it to explore three typical causes of imbalance (poor diet in Chapter 2.3, imbalance in emotions in Chapter 2.4, and unhealthy fascia in Chapter 2.5).

WHAT IS YOUR BODY CONSTITUTION TYPE?

B ody constitution is an integral and fundamental construct of TCM, as it lays the foundation for diagnosis, treatment, and disease prevention. Each individual's constitution is influenced by inherited factors and acquired factors (what happens to your body during your lifetime). Understanding your unique constitution will guide you toward making better lifestyle decisions.

However, while body constitution is a core TCM concept widely applied in daily practice, there are many debates and challenges surrounding the subjective nature of the diagnoses. In light of this, one of the major developments in TCM over the past three decades has been building a consistent classification of the body constitution types. One strategy was to develop a standardized and structured questionnaire that TCM practitioners can use.

Broader Application of the
Body Constitution Questionnaire

Since its creation, the body constitution questionnaire has been used by organi-
zations, practitioners, and online websites as a reference to one's constitution.
But again, the questionnaire is intended to be one of many diagnostic methods
used by TCM practitioners. For a more comprehensive assessment, please visit
your local TCM practitioner.

To start off this part of the book, we'd like you to complete this standard body constitution questionnaire. The version here is a translated
version by distinguished professor Qi Wang of the Beijing University
of Chinese Medicine. Professor Wang is the subject matter expert on
TCM body constitution, with many crediting him for creating a universal definition for TCM constitutions. The questionnaire that he created
is used by many TCM physicians around the world as part of the diagnosis and screening process. (His name "Qi" is pronounced the same
way as TCM Qi but isn't the same character.) You'll see a number of
tables on the following pages, each of which has six to eight statements
about different conditions related to physical or emotional health. For
each one, circle the number associated with the option that best applies
to you. Just go with your gut feeling to avoid spending too much time
per question.

When you're done with a table, tally up the scores, then determine
an average for the category and enter the number in the space provided.
At the end of the questionnaire, you can compare the scores of different
sections. The section with the highest score is your primary constitution. If you look at the pages following the questionnaire, you'll find
a brief description of each constitution type. Then in later chapters in
Part 2, we'll show you examples of how you can use knowledge of your

constitution type to help you identify imbalances and develop solutions to address those imbalances.

Using the Body Constitution Questionnaire

To illustrate how this works, the following table shows an excerpt of the evaluation by our case study subject Ben (you'll find his full questionnaire in Appendix E). As you can see, for the "Balanced Health" section of the questionnaire, he ended up with an average score of 2.43.

EXAMPLE OF A COMPLETED CONSTITUTION TABLE

Balanced Health	Never	Seldom	Sometimes	Frequent	Always
Easily fatigued	1	2	(3)	4	5
Weak/breathy voice	(1)	2	3	4	5
Constantly feeling down or gloomy	1	(2)	3	4	5
Cold aversion (including to AC or fans in summer)	(1)	2	3	4	5
Sensitive to natural changes in the environment (climate, weather)	1	2	3	(4)	5
Insomnia	1	(2)	3	4	5
Forgetful	1	2	3	(4)	5
Total score divided by 7: 2.43					

STEP 1: COMPLETE THE QUESTIONNAIRE

Work through each section of the following table and mark the answer that applies to you for each item. Calculate an average score for each section.

BODY CONSTITUTION QUESTIONNAIRE

QI DEFICIENCY

	Never	Seldom	Sometimes	Frequent	Always
Fatigued	1	2	3	4	5
Shortness of breath/panting (compared to people of your age)	1	2	3	4	5
Heart palpitations	1	2	3	4	5
Dizzy or lightheaded	1	2	3	4	5
Frequent colds and flu (especially when season changes)	1	2	3	4	5
Aloof and emotionally distant	1	2	3	4	5
Weak, breathy, or feeble voice	1	2	3	4	5
Excessive perspiration or night sweats	1	2	3	4	5
Total score divided by 8					

YANG DEFICIENCY

	Never	Seldom	Sometimes	Frequent	Always
Cold hands and feet/pale skin	1	2	3	4	5
Cold intolerance (sensitive to cold environments)	1	2	3	4	5
More layers of clothing than those around you	1	2	3	4	5
Chills in the abdomen, lower back, or knees	1	2	3	4	5
Prone to sickness/getting sick all the time (weak immune system)	1	2	3	4	5
Erectile dysfunction (male) or loss of sex drive (male or female)	1	2	3	4	5
Stomachache or diarrhea after eating cold/raw food and beverages	1	2	3	4	5
Repressed	1	2	3	4	5
Total score divided by 8					

YIN DEFICIENCY

	Never	Seldom	Sometimes	Frequent	Always
Warm or burning sensations in hands and feet (like to expose limbs or touch cool surfaces)	1	2	3	4	5
Feeling hot but no fever	1	2	3	4	5
Dry skin/cracked lips	1	2	3	4	5
Dark/burgundy-colored lips (natural state without makeup)	1	2	3	4	5
Constipation/dry hard stool	1	2	3	4	5
Redness/flushing of cheeks or face	1	2	3	4	5
Dry eyes	1	2	3	4	5
Dry mouth or constant thirst	1	2	3	4	5
Total score divided by 8					

PHLEGM-WETNESS

	Never	Seldom	Sometimes	Frequent	Always
Chest tightness/ abdominal bloating	1	2	3	4	5
Heaviness in limbs and body/lethargic	1	2	3	4	5
Delayed or slow bowel movements	1	2	3	4	5
Oily forehead	1	2	3	4	5
Puffy eyes	1	2	3	4	5
Mouth feels sticky	1	2	3	4	5
Excessive mucus in throat	1	2	3	4	5
Thick tongue coating	1	2	3	4	5
Total score divided by 8					

WETNESS-HEAT

	Never	Seldom	Sometimes	Frequent	Always
Oily face/nose	1	2	3	4	5
Prone to acne	1	2	3	4	5
Bitter/bad taste in mouth	1	2	3	4	5
Sticky stool/tenesmus (sensation of needing to pass stool)	1	2	3	4	5
Hot or burning urine/dark urine (dark like amber)	1	2	3	4	5
Yellow discharge (female only)	1	2	3	4	5
Sweaty testicles (male only)	1	2	3	4	5
Total score divided by 6					

BLOOD STASIS

	Never	Seldom	Sometimes	Frequent	Always
Petechiae/ecchymosis (unexplained bruising without bumping into things)	1	2	3	4	5
Rashes on face	1	2	3	4	5
Body aches	1	2	3	4	5
Dull skin tone	1	2	3	4	5
Dark circles under the eyes	1	2	3	4	5
Poor memory/forgetfulness	1	2	3	4	5
Dark red or purple lips (natural state without makeup)	1	2	3	4	5
Total score divided by 7					

QI STAGNATION

	Never	Seldom	Sometimes	Frequent	Always
Depressed or unmotivated	1	2	3	4	5
Anxiety/frustration	1	2	3	4	5
Emotional and sensitive	1	2	3	4	5
Easily frightened/fearful	1	2	3	4	5
Mastalgia (breast pain for women)/ discomfort around the sides of rib cage (both men and women)	1	2	3	4	5
Sighing	1	2	3	4	5
Sensation of lump in the throat	1	2	3	4	5
Total score divided by 7					

BALANCED HEALTH

	Never	Seldom	Sometimes	Frequent	Always
Easily fatigued	5	4	3	2	1
Weak/breathy voice	5	4	3	2	1
Constantly feeling down or gloomy	5	4	3	2	1
Cold aversion (including to AC or fans in summer)	5	4	3	2	1
Sensitive to natural changes in the environment (climate, weather)	5	4	3	2	1
Insomnia	5	4	3	2	1
Forgetful	5	4	3	2	1
Total score divided by 7					

STEP 2: COMPARE YOUR SCORES

When you're done with the questionnaire, copy the average score from each section into the following table.

BODY CONSTITUTION SUMMARY

Constitution	Average Score	
Qi Deficiency		
Yang Deficiency		
Yin Deficiency		
Phlegm-Wetness		
Wetness-Heat		
Blood Stasis		
Qi Stagnation		
Balanced Health		

The constitution with the highest number is your *primary* constitution. If you have two or more high scores that are the same, that means you have more than one predominant constitution (which is totally normal!).

STEP 3: INTERPRET THE RESULTS

Your basic body constitution type will have a big impact on each aspect of your strategies to achieve optimal fitness and health. The following table includes descriptions of each body constitution, so find the one (or more) that applies to you. Traditionally, TCM addresses nine classifications of body constitutions, but we have included only eight here. (The ninth type, commonly called "Special Conditions," deals mostly with issues related to your genetic inheritance and the care you received during the first four months of your life.)

CHARACTERISTICS OF THE CONSTITUTION TYPES

Neutral and Balanced Health • Physically fit • Emotionally stable • Healthy appetite • Adapts well to surroundings and climate changes	**Qi Deficiency** • Easily fatigued or out of breath • Susceptible to common cold or common flu • Sweats easily with little physical activity • Sensitive to changes in climate and season
Yang Deficiency • Aversion to cold and humid weather • Prone to water retention and diarrhea • Unwell after eating cold food • Prefers warm or hot drinks • Cold hands, feet, and abdomen	**Yin Deficiency** • Prefers cold drinks • Aversion to hot and dry weather • Warm at the palms of the hand and soles of the feet • Dry mouth, throat, or nose • Dry stools or constipation
Phlegm-Wetness • Oily face and forehead • Sluggish, chest tightness, and heaviness in the limbs • Uncomfortable in humid and rainy environments • Has a habit of consuming greasy food high in fats and sugar	**Wetness-Heat** • Oily face, prone to acne or pimples • Feeling fatigued or heaviness in the body • Easily agitated • Incomplete defecation, constipation, or dry stools • Excessive secretions at the reproductive organs
Blood Stasis • Forgetfulness • Irritable or easily agitated • Dull complexion and pigmentation on the skin • Prone to bleeding disorders • Susceptible to insomnia	**Qi Stagnation** • Prone to mood swings, anxiety, and depression • Excessive sighing or deep breaths • Tightness in chest • Adapts poorly to mental stimulation

How This Relates to You

Now that you have a general idea of your primary constitution, keep that in mind as you read through the other chapters in this part of the book. If you have two or more predominant constitutions, the goal is to help you understand the connection between them and, most important, to find the root cause of imbalances. All constitutions are linked together, and some may manifest with similar outward symptoms. Even if we discuss examples that do not match your constitutions exactly, pay attention to how body constitution can be used to identify challenges people face in meeting their health and fitness goals.

A Snapshot in Time

Remember that the scores you give yourself today might be different from the scores you would have given yourself yesterday or a week ago—and different from what you'd give yourself tomorrow or a week or a month or a year from tomorrow. Our body constitution changes from day to day and year to year according to our age and lifestyle. We encourage you to take this questionnaire from time to time to test for your constitution and help identify potential issues.

THE FACTORS THAT UPSET DYNAMIC BALANCE

The Western world rarely pays attention to dynamic balance in the sense that we have used in this book. Rather than looking for causes of imbalance, Western physicians tend to look for pathogens—anything (such as a virus) that causes a disease. TCM uses the term *pathogen* to refer to factors that affect the body's Qi and the balance of Yin and Yang. In other words, the primary focus of TCM theory is on the identification of general factors that are causing the deviation from the balanced state.

Ancient TCM physicians identified common factors in the body that led to imbalance. As you can see in the figure at the beginning of this chapter, the body can be pushed out of balance by both internal and external factors. Health can be affected by the climate, the season, the weather, your lifestyle, your emotions, and your amount of physical activity. In this chapter, we will explore the internal and external factors that may impact your overall health and athletic performance, using a case study to provide a point of reference.

Factors							
Internal				External			
Diet	Emotions	Constitution	Physical Health	Climate	Geographic Location	Season	

Case Study: Ben's Bulking Journey

Ben is a thirty-three-year-old investment banker from San Francisco. He is 5 feet, 11 inches tall and slender. Outside of his stressful work, he enjoys working out and playing basketball. Although Ben is not an elite athlete, his competitive spirit is second to none. Because of that, he has studied numerous books and internet videos on performance enhancement. In the spring of 2019, he decided to hire a personal trainer to help him reach his goals. He also decided to document his daily routine and workout progress on Instagram. Here is the exchange between the pair during the initial session:

> **Trainer:** Ben, you are too skinny. You will have to bulk up if you want to become a better athlete. You must become bigger, stronger, and faster. Plus, summer is coming up. Don't you want some blazing abs to show the world your dedication and transformation?
>
> **Ben:** I do! How should I go about building muscle mass?
>
> **Trainer:** First, you must put in the hard work at the gym. Then it is all about nutrition. You have got to hit your calories and macros. This is what you have to do:

- Drink black coffee or caffeinated drinks before
  the session to amp you up.

- Hit your daily 3,000-calorie target
  (his daily average is 2,500).

- Consume food every three hours.

- Have tons of lean protein.

- Eat brown rice instead of white rice.

- Drink plenty of milk.

- Consume healthy fats like avocado and nuts.

- Utilize protein shakes as snacks.

- Don't forget to eat your fruits and
  veggies along the way.

Ben: No offense, but this sounds so demotivating and difficult . . .

Trainer: Are *you* willing to dedicate some effort into becoming a better you? The hard days are the ones that make you stronger!

Ben: All right, I will have a go at this . . .

Since Ben is not a skillful cook, he would prepare a large batch of food at once, then divide it into smaller meals. Ben strictly followed the trainer's advice for three months, and his gains are summarized in the following table. As you can see, Ben gained weight and saw improvements in his one-repetition maximum (1RM) for squat, deadlift, and bench press.

BEN'S PROGRESS

	Weight	Squat 1RM	Deadlift 1RM	Bench Press 1RM
Start	164 lb.	100 kg	130 kg	60 kg
End	175 lb.	115 kg	150 kg	70 kg
Gain	+11 lb.	+15 kg	+20 kg	+10 kg

Trainer: Look, we have made significant progress. I am so proud of your effort!

Ben: Yeah, I look great now, but somehow, I am feeling a bit "off." I feel a bit tired and sluggish throughout the day, and I am struggling with constipation.

Trainer: Try consuming a cup of black coffee or some pre-workout supplements whenever you are struggling with motivation. Caffeine will make you feel more alert.

Ben: But I am already drinking three to four cups of coffee per day . . .

Ben's Problems

Ben's story is fictitious for the purposes of this book, but how many times have we heard of or experienced stories like Ben's? It appears that the objectives of the initial training session have been achieved—Ben gained some weight, and he could see better numbers for his bench press, squat, and deadlift. The problem though is that he did not *feel* stronger or faster. In fact, he felt bloated and sluggish, to the point where he had to consume two to three coffees throughout the day to stay alert. He also suffered from constipation. He took the questionnaire (you can find the full results in Appendix E). The following table shows the summary results. Ben indicated that his constitution is wetness-heat and Yin deficiency.

RESULTS FROM BEN'S CONSTITUTION QUESTIONNAIRE

Constitution	Ben's Numbers
Qi Deficiency	1.875
Yang Deficiency	1.25
Yin Deficiency	3.125
Phlegm-Wetness	2.75
Wetness-Heat	3.333
Blood Stasis	2.714
Qi Stagnation	1.429
Balanced Health	2.43

Feeling lethargic or sluggish is a common phenomenon in the fitness world, and it is a sign that the body is not able to maintain homeostasis.

There are three common causes of imbalance that TCM principles would lead Ben to explore:

1. A diet that is imbalanced compared to his body's needs

2. Emotions that are not properly managed, in that they have strayed too far into a particular direction (not necessarily negative, but positive too)

3. Unhealthy fascia, which compromises the body's movement and communication system

In the following chapters, we'll go through each of these factors, explain what balance and imbalance mean in TCM terms, and apply the thought process of TCM to see whether we can identify the culprit behind Ben's apparent physical gains but growing lethargy.

CHAPTER 2.3

AN IMBALANCE IN DIET DEPENDS ON YOUR SITUATION

T he view of a healthy diet in the United States has undergone significant transformation and progression as scientific research on human nutrition advances. While the objective of earlier nutritional research was to look for the "optimal" diet, recent findings suggest that one size doesn't fit all. Even the exact same diet followed by two individuals can produce varying outcomes. What is effective for one person might not be effective for another. Thus, the common consensus in the research community is that dieting plans must be individualized and case dependent. Turns out, the Chinese have been preaching this message for thousands of years.

The fundamental principle of TCM dietary practice is that an optimal universal diet does not exist. Unlike the seemingly esoteric and unquantifiable languages of TCM diagnostic practices, the TCM dietary philosophy is much easier to comprehend and digest (pun intended). In Part 1, we explained the essential concepts in TCM—body constitution, the Yin-Yang philosophy, Zang-Fu (the five organs), and the five phases. Together with the five flavors, which we'll explain in this chapter, these concepts are used to determine the best foods for an individual.

Although the US and Chinese cultures have distinctly different understandings of nutrition and dieting practices, the two can coexist and complement each other. Blending the best of Eastern and Western traditions means that an athlete can adopt a comprehensive, systematic, and holistic approach to decipher which diet plan best fits them. The following table compares the primary language used in the East and the West.

EAST VS. WEST VIEW OF DIET

East	West
Focused on the overall effects	Focused on individual components
Qi	Carbohydrates
Body Constitution	Protein
Yin-Yang (Cold-Hot)	Fat
Five Phases	Vitamins
Five Flavors	Minerals
Food Nature	

The Gut and the Brain

Despite the phrase *gut feeling* that implicitly connects the gut and the brain, what happens in the gut (digestion) and brain (emotions) have been studied and treated separately in Western medicine. Dr. Emeran Mayer, a gastroenterologist (doctors who are trained to diagnose and treat problems in the digestive tract) and a professor of medicine at the University of California, Los Angeles, published a fascinating book, *The Mind-Gut Connection*, that explores the ways that the gut and the brain communicate. Referencing recent scientific findings that the gut and the brain are intricately linked, Mayer touches on how dietary habits may impact gut-brain communication. He also shares valuable stories on how a better gut can lead to improvements in the brain.

Balancing the Five Flavors

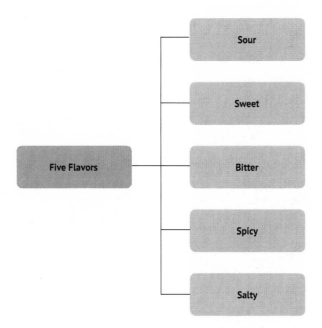

Flavor is a critical part of any diet. The Chinese have distilled all the flavors into five categories, known as the five flavors—sour, sweet, bitter, spicy, and salty. While these flavors are similar to those that we perceive on our palate, flavors in TCM are used to communicate the therapeutic effect that each taste encompasses. So it isn't just the flavor itself that is important but how the body reacts to the flavor. Each flavor is associated with a specific organ, season, and type of energy (Qi). Food can restore imbalances for individual body constitutions, while it can also exacerbate any problems with the body. The flavor of food plays a critical role in our health and body function. The Chinese even believe that particular flavor cravings are signals of need.

Ancient View of the Flavors

Each flavor governs a part of the metabolic process. These basic tastes that are naturally contained in foods were first recorded in *The Yellow Emperor's Classic of Medicine,* a text dating from the third century BC. In most TCM historical herb books, taste was often the first property of an herb to be mentioned.

Have you ever wondered why some people prefer spicy food, while others prefer salty or sweet foods? If every flavor is associated with a particular type of energy, you craving that flavor implies that your body wants it: Sour craving is a signal of emotional or physical stagnation. Bitter craving is a sign that we are feeling down or emotional. Spicy craving is a need for heat, as it is related to the immune system. Salty craving may indicate that there are problems with kidney and urinary bladder health. Sweet craving, a popular yet guilty craving in the modern world, is the body requesting energy.

The five flavors' association with the five phases and seasons is summarized in the following table.

OVERVIEW OF THE FIVE FLAVORS

	Flavor				
	Sour	**Bitter**	**Sweet**	**Spicy**	**Salty**
Zang-Fu (Organs)	Liver (Zang) Gallbladder (Fu)	Heart (Zang) Small Intestine (Fu)	Spleen (Zang) Stomach (Fu)	Lung (Zang) Large Intestine (Fu)	Kidney (Zang) Bladder (Fu)
Phase	Wood	Fire	Earth	Metal	Water
Flavor Action	Stimulates contraction and absorption	Disperses heat; drains and dries	Moistens and nourishes	Disperses stagnation and promotes circulation	Softens and moves downward
Season	Spring	Summer	Late Summer/ Transition between seasons	Autumn	Winter

The theory of the five phases establishes relationships between organs, flavors, seasons, and emotions. Each flavor corresponds to Zang-Fu organs and has a therapeutic action on Qi and blood. Now, flavor action may or may not work to your advantage. Because of the association, a particular flavor may help correct an imbalance or do the direct opposite—exacerbate it. Knowing your body constitution, you can begin to think about whether your diet is enhancing or impeding your performance.

Flavors: Finding a Balance?

In keeping with the theme of this book, the challenge for each of us is to maintain a balance of flavors in our diet. Having the right amount of each flavor can
help our bodies cope not just with athletic performance but with everything
that happens in life. Appendix C includes a table that shows what can happen
if you have too much, too little, or the right amount of the flavors in your diet.
And later, we'll go into more detail about how you can analyze your own diet
and adjust the flavor balance to suit your body constitution, season, and so on.

Sugar: Enemy or Friend?

Of all the flavors, the one that is discussed the most is "sweet" and
especially sugar cravings. Is sugar detrimental to athletic performance?
Among the fitness community, there is almost a sense of guilt that
comes with craving sugar. In a modern culture inundated by added
sugar, it may be difficult to imagine how sweets can benefit health. But
the truth is, certain kinds and adequate amounts of sweets are essential
to sustaining life. Again, let's take a step back and examine different
perspectives on the topic.

ENERGY PRODUCTION BASICS FROM
WESTERN PHYSIOLOGY

Open any credible textbook on health and wellness and you should find
sections or chapters on energy production. Humans need energy to perform biological work (such as physical activity), like how a car needs gas
for it to move. And every athlete's performance depends greatly on how
well they manage their diet to generate the kinds of energy needed for
their sport or activity—which means athletes must have a basic understanding of the mechanisms in which energy is produced in the body.

You may have heard of adenosine triphosphate (ATP), the molecule that functions as the energy currency of cells because of its key role in metabolism and energy transfer. And although there is a minimal amount of ATP stored in the muscles, the majority of ATP is synthesized from the diet, from the macronutrients—carbohydrates, protein, and fats, which are converted into usable energy.

There are three primary energy systems in the human body to replenish ATP—the phosphagen system, fast glycolysis, and the oxidative system. The three systems can be considered a continuum, as they will all be recruited to generate energy for the body to function as exercise duration increases: The phosphagen system powers the initial contraction of a muscle, which next draws on fast glycolysis and then eventually the oxidative system the longer the muscle needs to work. But different parts of the system will become predominant depending on the needs of the physical activity.

The main characteristics of the three systems are shown in the following chart adapted from *Essentials of Strength Training and Conditioning*, published by the National Strength and Conditioning Association.

ENERGY SYSTEMS

Energy System	Phosphagen System	Fast Glycolysis	Oxidative System
Duration	< 6 seconds	30 seconds to 2 minutes	> 3 minutes
Characteristics	Used for short, explosive movements	For movements that last more than 6 seconds	Used for movements longer than 3 minutes
Fuel Source	Creatine phosphate	Glycogen	Free fatty acids when resting; during exercise, carbohydrates, fats when glycogen sparing, and protein as a last resort

These three bioenergy systems have a profound impact on human performance, health, and longevity.

If we look into the fuel sources of the systems, glycogen is an essential fuel source for movements that are longer than six seconds (which in many sports happens frequently). Glycogen is the stored form of glucose in the body, and glucose is a simple sugar (monosaccharide). The primary function of sugar is to provide *energy* to power your activities. This would also explain why carbohydrates are critical to everyday functioning. Carbohydrates are mostly made up of either simple sugars (glucose, fructose, and sucrose) or complex sugars (long sugar chains). Therefore, sugar is a vital source of energy even if it is promoted as the devil that everyone should avoid. Naturally occurring sugars have essential nutrients that are vital to maintaining good health and good athletic performance, so these should be a staple in an athlete's diet. Nonetheless, refined sugar consumption should be minimized.

Spitting Out Your Sports Drink?

A trendy practice that exemplifies the power of taste is the practice of spitting out a carbohydrate sports drink (usually sweet in taste) after swishing it around in the mouth. Studies have shown that this practice may result in improved performance, while the mechanism behind why this is happening is not yet fully understood. Since there are many receptors in the mouth that are sending direct signals to the brain, one possible explanation is that swishing the carbohydrate drink essentially tricks the mind into thinking that there is more energy on the way, which results in improved performance. How cool is that?

SWEET TASTE FROM A TCM PERSPECTIVE

When TCM principles were first being developed, the Chinese did not have the technology to explore the bioenergetic systems. Through years of observation and practice, it is recorded that the sweet flavor nourishes the spleen and stomach, which have functions that revolve around digestion and absorption of nutrients, thus giving the body *energy*. The sweet flavor also helps to lubricate the body by replenishing deficient Qi, soothing the mind, and generating body fluid.

Added sweets were rare in native Chinese culture. The sweet-tasting foods in Chinese culture were usually starches and meats (yes, meat like chicken and pork have natural sweetness in them even if you do not marinate them in a sweet sauce). It might be stretching one's imagination to categorize those foods as sweet by the modern definition for sweetness. Yet our taste threshold for sweetness is blinded by all the added sugars (like corn syrup) in the modern lifestyle.

PIECING TOGETHER THE EASTERN AND WESTERN VIEWS OF SUGAR

Although the two perspectives use different language to express energy production, they both would agree that sugar gives humans energy. This gives us an interesting insight as to why we crave sweets whenever we are working, studying, or exercising: We need energy. Dr. Richard Johnson, author of *The Sugar Fix*, even argues that craving sugar is a biological survival mechanism: Those who ate sugar were more likely to survive. Thus, you crave sweets because sweets have been an ever-present part of human history. The problem of modern society is that our diet is inundated with sugar. Therefore, we say that you should reach for a balanced point where you are eating enough sugar to fuel energy but not so much that there is too much sweetness in your diet.

Nature of Food

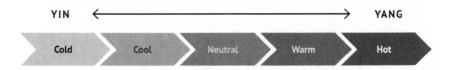

YIN ←————————————————————→ YANG

| Cold | Cool | Neutral | Warm | Hot |

The flavors of a food are only part of the picture. As you have probably experienced yourself, different foods elicit different responses and sensations from the body. The concept of Yin-Yang (Chapter 1.2) can also be applied to food. In TCM, food is measured on a spectrum, from cold to hot. Cold and cool are symbolized by Yin, whereas warm and hot are Yang because of the opposing nature. *The nature of food is not determined by its actual temperature but rather by the effects the food has on the body after consumption.* If you eat foods that are predominantly cooling in nature, such as salad and clams, your body will produce more Yin energy: slower-moving and colder. Conversely, if you eat foods that are predominantly warming in nature, such as lamb and ginger, your body will produce more Yang energy: faster-moving and hotter.

To understand the logic behind the nature of food, we first must understand how food is classified. Here is the general rule of thumb in determining the type of energy:

- If it grows in the earth and darkness: Yin/Cool
- If it grows in the air and sunshine: Yang/Warm
- If it is soft, wet, and cool: Yin/Cool
- If it is hard, dry, and spicy: Yang/Warm

The way that the food is cooked may also change its nature. If you are cooking lettuce (which is cool in nature), steaming, poaching, and boiling helps preserve its cool nature. Deep-frying, stir-frying, and roasting change the nature of food to be warmer. That's why foods that are deep-fried, stir-fried, or roasted are considered warming foods in TCM. Keep in mind that the Chinese classified the nature of food through trial and error. It was a long learning process as Chinese physicians observed ulcers, headaches, constipation, and other body signals that human bodies gave when they were out of balance. For this reason, the Chinese understood clearly that the reaction to food and medicine varies by the individual, and a one-size-fits-all methodology does not exist. This would also explain why people disagree on the nature of a certain food, because the effects of the food vary from person to person. The nature of common foods according to the TCM system is listed in Appendix C.

SEASONAL CONDITIONS AND DIET

TCM is sometimes viewed as superstitious when practitioners associate seasons with energy. But think of the last freezing weather that you had to endure and the urge to remain in bed, then compare that with a sunny summer day when you were crushing your workout session or meeting friends at an outdoor coffee shop. You felt different in those different conditions, right?

The Chinese strive to live in harmony with the world, which means eating foods that can help us cope with the different seasons. The following table shows how the seasons relate to flavors and other TCM concepts.

THE CONNECTION BETWEEN SEASONS AND OTHER TCM CONCEPTS

Season	Phase	Properties	Zang-Fu	Flavor
Spring	Wood	Time of birth and new beginnings	Liver/ Gallbladder	Sour
Summer	Fire	Active, warming, and dynamic	Heart/Small Intestine	Bitter
Late Summer (or the time in between seasons)	Earth	A time of stabilization and transition	Spleen/ Stomach	Sweet
Autumn	Metal	A time of harvest, shorter days, and preparations for winter	Lung/ Colon	Spicy
Winter	Water	A time of cooling, storing, and resting	Kidney/ Bladder	Salty

GEOGRAPHICAL LOCATION

Long before the globalization of food, our diets were hugely decided by our geographical location. This is exemplified by the Eskimos, the Indigenous people living in the Arctic regions of the world: Their diets are high in protein and fat. If this diet is followed elsewhere, the person is essentially begging for heart disease. Yet early studies have found that the Eskimos have low rates of heart disease—which has become a fascinating topic for many researchers.

The TCM view on this matter is simple: The Eskimos are required to have a diet high in protein and fats by nature. They do not have access to fresh vegetables and carbohydrates that someone from a tropical area would typically have. Therefore, the diet that is accessible to the Eskimos is suitable for them.

The same can be said about other regions of the world. Foods that are grown locally are designed for you to eat. Our diet should be in harmony with the surrounding environment. Blindly following diets that are vastly different from the current environment is insidious and unnatural.

What About Coffee?

No modern book about diet can avoid the topic of coffee. It has taken the world by storm. It is not an expensive item (other than some prestigious beans), tastes great, and has caffeine, which keeps our minds awake, fresh, and ready to conquer the challenging tasks ahead of us.

From a Western health perspective, coffee seems to be a double-edged sword. On the one hand, coffee contains antioxidants. On the other, high consumption of caffeinated coffee can lead to negative effects, such as headaches, an increase in blood pressure, and mental health issues (restlessness, anxiety, insomnia).

What about from a TCM perspective? Is coffee healthy? Let's explore together using what we know so far. To start, you will first have to know that what we call a coffee bean is the seed of a coffee fruit (or coffee cherry/coffee berry because of its appearance) from a coffee plant. A coffee fruit starts out green before turning red (or other colors depending on the variety) as it ripens. And that is when the fruit, then subsequently the seed, is picked from the coffee plant. Since it grows from the ground, the fruit and its seed would originally be considered a cool food in TCM. But before you put the bag of coffee beans that you purchased into the filter, or the espresso machine, the batches of seeds inside the fruit must be roasted. The level of roasting affects how the beans taste and smell. After roasting, the most common taste is bitterness.

We now know that roasting changes a food that is cool in nature to warm in nature. Foods that are warm in nature stimulate Qi and blood, and coffee certainly stimulates Qi and blood by giving us energy. And for the bitter taste, it is beneficial to clear out dampness and heat. All of those are positive aspects of drinking coffee.

Is coffee for everyone? So far, we have shared that a diet should take into consideration the food's or drink's Yin-Yang nature and the flavors, plus a person's body constitution, geographical location, and season in which they are ingesting that delicious food or drink. Given what we know so far, coffee may be most beneficial to those who live in a damp environment looking for an energy boost.

But then why is there a Starbucks coffee shop in every corner of the world? While it is true that Starbucks has a top-notch team of business executives that built the empire, the expansion would not have been possible if Starbucks hadn't become popular in Seattle back in the 1970s. If you examine the region closely, coffee is a great drink for Seattleites. Geographically, the Pacific Northwest has damp weather, and damp weather creates dampness in the body. Coffee (black coffee), being bitter, can clear dampness from the body, and it provides a boost in energy, making it a perfect drink for residents in the area.

However, just because coffee is great for Seattleites doesn't mean that coffee is good for you as an individual, no matter where you live. Take into consideration your constitution, geographical location, and climate to decipher whether coffee is a good fit for you. Even if coffee is a suitable drink for your current circumstances, remember that too much bitter flavor can injure the heart and bones (there is research that links excessive caffeine and bone loss). Also remember that coffee is a double-edged sword. What is the key in handling a double-edged sword? Balance.

Action Steps: Variety, Constitution, and Climate

For decades, health authorities and schools have educated us to eat balanced meals that incorporate foods from different groups. Even within the same groups—such as grains, vegetables, and fruits—we are encouraged to include a variety of selections to ensure adequate nutritional intake. Each food offers a unique blend of nutrients, so cycling through different foods is a good way to ensure that an athlete is covering all the bases.

Another strategy for selecting food according to the body is to pick foods that do not significantly alter the balance of Yin-Yang. Take a person with a predominant wetness-heat body type, for example: Eating foods that are warm in nature would exacerbate the current problem. Instead, the person should consume foods that will help them return to a balanced state. The same train of thought can be applied to the climate.

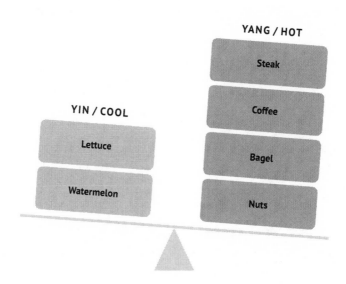

A Yang-dominant diet tilts the body to a Yang state.

BEN'S CASE STUDY:
DIET OF IMMODERATION

Like Ben, many athletes go on different diets depending on their training phases and goals. To sustain dynamic balance, the Chinese emphasized the importance of harmony between one's constitution, the five flavors, the nature of food, and the geography and climate of an area. The following characteristics are all needed to assess whether a diet is in harmony.

- Constitution
- Food flavor
- Food nature
- Season
- Geographical location
- Climate
- Food variety

Let's analyze Ben's diet as an example, but first, here's some important background information to consider:

- He has a thin body type that he's trying to bulk up.
- He lives in San Francisco, where the climate is warm and humid in the spring.
- He has a stressful daytime job.

Ben recorded his three-day bulking diet (target of 3,000 calories per day), which we've shown in the following table. You don't need to remember the details, but try to pay attention to the kinds of flavors he is including in his diet.

BEN'S DIET

Day 1: Wednesday

7:30 a.m.	4-egg omelet with spinach and cheese / 1 bagel / 1 cup of whole milk
9:00 a.m.	1 glass of iced black coffee
10:00 a.m.	Mass-gainer shake
12:30 p.m.	Pan-fried double chicken breast / Boiled broccoli with salt / Brown rice / Iced black coffee
3:00 p.m.	Roasted mixed nuts / Banana
4:00 p.m.	Pan-fried small chicken breast / Boiled broccoli / Brown rice
7:00 p.m.	Pan-fried sirloin steak / Stir-fried vegetables / Baked potato
9:30 p.m.	Casein protein shake / 1 cup of whole milk

Day 2: Thursday

8:00 a.m.	Sausage, egg, and cheese bagel / 1 large latte
10:00 a.m.	Mass-gainer shake
12:30 p.m.	Pan-fried double chicken breast / Boiled broccoli with salt / Brown rice / Iced black coffee
3:00 p.m.	Roasted mixed nuts / Banana
4:00 p.m.	Pan-fried small chicken breast / Boiled broccoli / Brown rice
7:00 p.m.	Pan-fried salmon / Stir-fried vegetables / Baked potato
9:30 p.m.	Casein protein shake / 1 cup of whole milk

Day 3: Friday

8:00 a.m.	Bacon, egg, and cheese bagel / 1 large latte
10:00 a.m.	Mass-gainer shake
12:30 p.m.	Pan-fried double chicken breast / Boiled broccoli with salt / Baked potato / Iced black coffee
3:00 p.m.	Banana and peanut butter sandwich
5:00 p.m.	Mixed nuts
7:30 p.m.	Chicken burrito with medium spicy salsa / Salad / Chips and guacamole
9:30 p.m.	Casein protein shake / 1 cup of whole milk

ANALYSIS OF BEN'S DIET

Let's analyze Ben's diet through the lens of what we have learned so far:

What is the current season?	Spring
Which city/town are you in?	San Francisco
What is the climate?	The temperature is in the mid-70s (about 23 degrees Celsius). Humidity is around 80%.

We went through Ben's diet and labeled each item according to both its flavor and nature. The following table shows an excerpt of our analysis (the full details are in Appendix E).

CLASSIFYING BEN'S DIET (EXCERPT)

Time	Contents	Flavor	Nature
5:00 p.m.	Pan-fried small chicken breast	Sweet, Salty	Warm
	Boiled broccoli with salt	Sweet, Salty	Cool

A summary of our analysis is shown in the following table.

SUMMARY ANALYSIS OF BEN'S DIET

	FLAVOR					NATURE Yin ⟷ Yang				
	Sour	Sweet	Bitter	Spicy	Salty	Cold	Cool	Neutral	Warm	Hot
Day 1	0	17	2	0	7	0	4	8	6	3
Day 2	0	14	2	0	9	0	3	8	7	3
Day 3	0	12	2	0	8	0	4	8	6	5
TOTAL	0	43	6	0	24	0	11	24	19	11

What common themes do you see in the analysis of Ben's diet? Write down your observations:

_____

_____

_____

_____

GIVE YOUR DIGESTIVE SYSTEM A BREAK, BEN!

When looking at the flavor and nature of Ben's diet, the first thing that jumped out to us was that it was dominated by the sweet flavor. The number of sweets would sometimes double the closest number, which was salty. Ben also rarely had spicy or sour foods. In terms of food nature, Ben's diet was more warm/hot than cool/cold.

And even without looking at the numbers, Ben's diet looks uninspiring—and so boring that it would be hard to sustain. Perhaps because Ben did not have the time or interest to cook, his food choices were quite limited. But he definitely scores low on variety in his diet!

Looking at Ben's scores, we can reach the following conclusions:

- The nature of his food indicates a Yin deficiency (no cold and relatively few cool foods). This could explain why Ben feels hot, is constipated, and is constantly thirsty.

- The flavors indicate wetness-heat (because of the heavy emphasis on sweet flavors). This contributes to why Ben feels bloated and lethargic, has slow bowel movements, and has an oily forehead.

The key issue is that the fluid in Ben's body is not distributed where it needs to be, and his diet is contributing to that imbalance. This links back to our core concept that we must look at the whole body to understand what is going on. The heat he has is a result of a lack in water (or Yin)—like how a forest fire starts in a dry autumn. The wetness however cannot moisten this heat, since it is more like tar oil than clear, cool water. Or think about what happens when oil or sugar is burned—it usually leaves a sticky stain and is hard to clean. "Greasy" and "sweet" avocados and nuts *when overconsumed* also leave a "sticky stain" on our "pot" (the spleen). This further suppresses the spleen's normal functions and is manifested in irregular stool patterns and low energy levels.

Now let's dissect his diet habits. Ben eats a lot of protein and drinks a lot of coffee, and his diet is dominated by the sweet flavor. In TCM, protein powder is considered to be hot in nature (Yang) because it is processed and has very little water retained (compared to the protein-water ratio in natural food). Imagine Ben putting all of these highly concentrated energy cubes into his body: What do you think happens? All the cells in his digestive system and the gut bacteria have to work out how to break down those big loads of protein into pieces.

Coffee is also roasted and concentrated, which makes it hot in nature as well. Remember the Starbucks story, where we said coffee is beneficial in humid climates because bitter clears out heat and dampness? This holds true for Ben's story, except he is having too much!

Also, having too much protein in a diet further burdens the spleen's digestive functions, as proteins are less efficient to break down for energy compared to starch.

When a food cannot be dissolved in water easily, it's considered to be relatively harder for the body to break down (since our body is 70% water, and water is the largest medium for metabolism). To break down these components, more energy is required by the body.

To make things worse, the way Ben processes his food is mostly by pan-frying and baking. This further reduces the amount of water retained in the food. Brown rice compared to white rice contains less water as well.

Let's assume that our body can have only a limited amount of energy each day, so overconsuming of such foods is like a company giving all the resources to just one department to handle a hard task. This leaves the other departments in the body with a minimal amount of energy, thus explaining why Ben feels tired and lethargic. Moreover, water in the body is all drawn to digest these warm-nature foods, causing the body to suffer from a hydro-imbalance. This explains his constant thirst, irregular stool patterns, and feeling hot but with no actual fever. Imbalance in water-oil ratio on the skin makes him more prone to acne and having excessive oil excretion. The water in his body is all used to compensate for his "dry" diet. This explains why he can be having wetness-heat and also Yin deficiency at the same time.

One last factor is Ben's radical shift in diet based on his trainer's advice, which caused an extra burden on his digestive system. Let's assume he normally ate three meals a day and maybe a snack on occasion. After the shift, he went to consuming seven meals a day. That is twice what his body is normally used to.

Imagine, out of nowhere, your boss tells you that he wants to expand the business tomorrow, so starting this week, you are all going to do twice the amount of work with the same pay. How would that make you feel? That is how the spleen, stomach, and digestive system felt when Ben had this sudden change in diet.

In TCM, the spleen is in charge of the body's digestion. It transforms the food we consume into nutrients and nourishes the body. Now it's working overtime with no breaks in between. It doesn't have the time and luxury to break down the food into fine components for better absorption. This lowers the energy efficiency in the food we take in. In the short run, it does seem to make our body look bulkier, but in the long run, our spleen's function is actually suffering, giving us less energy.

Fixing Ben's Diet Problems

To fix Ben's diet issues and to test out our hypothesis, Ben should try to do the following:

1. Cut the protein shakes entirely (because of all the added sugar and protein) and replace them with lean whole protein (such as fish).
2. Have no more than one cup of coffee per day.
3. Keep the number of meals but consume smaller portions for each meal to keep him energetic.

In short, Ben needs to give his digestive functions a break!

We'll have you do a more detailed analysis of your own diet later in this book (see Chapter 4.2), but for now, jot down some notes about what you think you're going to find and what ideas from this chapter you'd like to try for your own diet.

Notes on Your Diet

_____

_____

_____

_____

_____

_____

CONSIDER THE BALANCE OF YOUR EMOTIONS

We don't have to tell you that emotions affect physical performance and vice versa. You've probably had experiences where something good was happening in your life and you channeled that positive energy into your sport or activity, or where you were struggling with some aspect of your life and had difficulty maintaining focus and generating energy while working out or competing in a sport. Or where a strong physical performance helped raise your emotions and a bad performance brought on negative feelings.

We have been championing the idea throughout this book that the body and mind cannot be treated separately. Perhaps nowhere is that message clearer than when it comes to thinking about how emotions contribute to balance and imbalance in our bodies. What TCM adds to this area is a language and framework to better understand and explain those connections so we have more tools for maintaining dynamic balance.

The TCM Understanding of Emotions

The connection between emotions and bodily health was established thousands of years ago. Chen Wuzhe, a famous TCM practitioner in the Song dynasty (960–1279), proposed that emotions might lead to disharmony of the internal organs and then be reflected outwardly. He further divided emotions into seven categories, known as the seven emotions (the number seven can be thought of as a sacred number, holding special meaning in Chinese and Hindu traditions). The seven emotions are further categorized according to their Yin-Yang nature (calmness vs. energetic, as an example) and their effects on the movement of Qi. The following table lists the seven emotions as described in *The Yellow Emperor's Classic of Medicine*.

EMOTIONS AS VIEWED IN TCM

Emotion	Yin-Yang	Governed by	Movement of Qi	Symptoms of Excess
Anger	Yang	Liver	Rises	• Headaches • Dizziness • Forgetfulness • Tensed muscles
Joy	Yang	Heart	Slows	• Insomnia • Disorientation
Worry/Pensiveness	Yin	Spleen	Stagnates	• Bloating • Loss of appetite • Poor concentration • Menstrual cycle disruption
Anxiety	Yin	Lungs	Stagnates	• Gasping • Tight sensation in chest • Constipation • Fatigue
Melancholy/Grief/Sadness	Yin	Lungs	Depletes	• Shortness of breath • Congested nose • Muscle spasms • Rib cage pain
Fear	Yin	Kidney	Descends	• Urinary incontinence • Muscle atrophy • Hair loss • Pain in bones and joints • Erectile dysfunction
Fright	Yang	Kidney	Scatters	• Indecisiveness • Palpitations • Feeling stunned • Insane behavior

The categories of emotion are closely related to an individual's psychological and physiological state, as governed by the Zang-Fu, Qi, blood, and Yin-Yang. Our unconscious likes or dislikes toward the environment or situations in life can create excessive emotions, and this disruption challenges our ability to cope. It can disrupt our Qi, blood, meridians, and Zang-Fu, which can lead to further discomforts in the body. Ultimately, these deficiencies are detrimental to performance and everyday function.

This explains why, when an athlete encounters abrupt environmental changes or when they are under prolonged distress and emotional stimulations, their body's ability to maintain balance will be disrupted, and certain emotions will be in an excessive state.

Although each emotion is governed predominantly by one organ, the interconnectedness between the organs leads to feedback or compounding effects, as shown in the following figure. Strong emotions can affect our organs, which affects Qi. Or the reverse can happen: An imbalance in Qi can affect the organs, which affects our emotions.

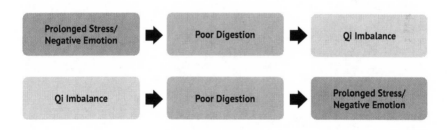

The connectedness of emotions, organs, and Qi

As an example, let's take a look at an emotion that many of us experience regularly—anger. Anger is governed by the liver. The liver has some important functions, such as regulating emotions; connecting the tendons, nails, and eyes; and assisting the digestive function of the spleen and the stomach.

When the liver Qi flows smoothly, our emotional status will be calm and peaceful, and the liver can do its job of aiding digestion via the spleen and stomach. But a strong emotion like anger can disrupt that flow, which leads to poor liver function. Or, if the liver Qi accumulates rather than continuing its flow, we can become hot-tempered and infuriated.

With either pathway, the result is the same. An excessive liver Qi gives an uprising force to the Qi in our body and manifests externally through physical symptoms such as dizziness and body aches. Plus, because the liver has an effect on the spleen and stomach, we can experience digestive issues such as a change in appetite as well.

As a final note, remember that the term *organ* in TCM theory has a broader implication than in Western medicine, referring not just to the physical organ itself but also to the functions of that organ.

Positive vs. Negative Emotions

"Don't worry, be happy." That refrain from a popular '80s song still resonates with people today. We are constantly being encouraged to avoid negative emotions and focus on positive emotions. As you can probably predict, the view that positive equals good and negative equals bad is not consistent with the TCM view of balance. There is a degree of negativity in positivity, and there is a degree of positivity in negativity. (Sound familiar? That's right, the two fishes in the Tai Chi symbol and the Yin-Yang philosophy!)

THE NEGATIVE IN THE POSITIVE: CAN YOU BE TOO HAPPY?

Happiness is a good thing, right? It's a positive emotion that helps us feel better. But Shigehiro Oishi, Ed Diener, and Richard Lucas published an analysis in 2007 titled "The Optimum Level of Well-Being:

Can People Be Too Happy?" They argued that "although happiness has positive consequences in general, being happier is not always better. Once a moderate level of happiness is achieved, further increases can be detrimental." They supported their claims by reporting empirical findings from different research studies.

Along the same train of thought, cognitive neuroscientist Tali Sharot delivered a TED Talk on how when we become unrealistically optimistic, we become biased, are more likely to engage in risky behaviors, and are prone to making poor decisions. Although positive emotions are generally constructive, too much produces negative consequences. In other words, we don't make the most rational decisions when we are overly happy. Thus, although positive emotions are an integral part of a happy and fulfilled life, it is fair to say that there must be a degree of negativity even in positivity.

THE POSITIVE IN THE NEGATIVE: FIGHT-OR-FLIGHT RESPONSE

Although negative emotions are generally perceived as destructive, there comes a time when these emotions can have a positive outcome. Take stress, for example. Stress leads to what we would normally characterize as negative emotions, including anxiety and worry. Does that mean all stress is bad?

Stress can be both emotional and physical; it prepares our body to act on a specific stimulus. One of the most common effects of stress is triggering what's known as the fight-or-flight response. Think about it: When our ancestors were exposed to a dangerous or life-threatening predator, they had to be ready to perform, whether that meant fighting the ferocious predator or running away.

From a physiological perspective, when the fight-or-flight response is triggered, a flood of hormones boosts the body's alertness and heart rate, sending extra blood to the muscles. The breathing rate increases so that more oxygen can be delivered to the brain. The liver will also produce glucose for more energy. Stress is, in short, part of our survival mechanism. And that is surely a positive thing.

Butterflies in the Stomach?

A large number of recent studies and books have identified a bidirectional communication between our brain, the gut, and the microorganisms that live in the digestive tracts. When Dr. Michael Gershon's book—*The Second Brain*—came out in 1998, it sparked much speculation about the abilities of the gut, which he called the second brain.

He pointed out that the gut had far greater influence on the body than just digestion. The gut influences our mental state and plays a key role in certain diseases throughout the body. In the previous chapter, we mentioned the term *gut feeling* and its implicit connection between the gut and the brain. Let's think about how that connection can manifest in our bodies.

We all have had the sensation of "butterflies in the stomach" before significant events. This is a classic example of how the brain and the gut are connected. The activation of the fight-or-flight response tones down or even switches off non-vital bodily processes, such as digestion, to redirect energy and blood flow to the muscles and the lungs, leading to that "fluttery" sensation in the gut. In short, the main processes behind the digestive system are inhibited, or turned off, when you are in a fight-or-flight state.

As it turns out, emotions like fear and anxiety prime our bodies to act and therefore are a critical aspect of sports performance and everyday function. To echo the words of psychology professor David Barlow, a past president of the American Psychological Association's Division of Clinical Psychology: "Without anxiety, little would be accomplished. The performance of athletes, entertainers, executives, artisans, and students would suffer; creativity would diminish; crops might not be planted. And we would all achieve that idyllic state long sought after in our fast-paced society of whiling away our lives under a shade tree. This would be as deadly for the species as nuclear war."[2] Barlow is well known for his contributions to the causes and treatment of anxiety disorders. Even he would admit that an adequate amount of anxiety is an essential part of life. Thus, what is typically known as a negative emotion can indeed have a positive impact.

Emotions and Dynamic Balance

When you have a dynamic balance in your emotions, you will still experience both positive and negative emotions, sometimes in the extreme. You cannot have an absence of either type of emotion because then there would be no balance: no Yin for the Yang or vice versa. The problem, rather, comes from an inordinate amount of either positive or negative emotions.

As we've discussed, though the fight-or-flight response was designed to quickly ignite the turbo systems of our engines, the engine should not be on for extended periods of time nor be constantly triggered for nonthreatening situations. What do our engines do when we are stuck in traffic, when we are scrolling through social media, when we are busy working the whole day, or much worse, when we experience the self-destructive doubt of whether we have what it takes to perform at our best? Our engines are tricked into fight-or-flight mode because suddenly we turn these everyday situations into a perceived life-threatening situation. And that's not good.

In their *New York Times* bestselling book *How to Perform Under Pressure: The Science of Doing Your Best When It Matters Most*, psychologists Hendrie Weisinger and J. P. Pawliw-Fry share some fascinating

2   Barlow, D. H. 1988. *Anxiety and Its Disorders: The Nature and Treatment of Anxiety and Panic.* New York: The Guilford Press.

insights on managing emotions under pressure situations. One strategy is to understand the difference between "I need" and "I want." The moment that you see the *need* to react quickly—not just some action that you *want* to take—your brain turns on the fight-or-flight turbo system because you think the issue now threatens your life in some way. Maybe your salary will be affected if you arrive late. Maybe you think the only way to be likable is to be hyperconnected on social media. Maybe you think that the upcoming game will define your abilities as an athlete. See where we are going with this? Our bodies can overreact to stressors that are not life-threatening.

Because our digestive system is temporarily turned off during fight-or-flight situations, prolonged overreaction (stress) can cause sustained blockage. It is common for people who are chronically stressed to experience symptoms such as diarrhea or constipation. Therefore, *the effects of your diet and your emotions are inextricably linked.* These types of non-life-threatening stimuli, if ill-managed, can be mentally draining and exhausting.

Every one of us will encounter serious stressors at some point in our lives: health problems, family crises, job or housing concerns. Dealing with these actual fight-or-flight situations is normal, though you should still strive for a balance in which no negative emotions take over your life for a prolonged period. But for the purposes of this book, what we want to help you recognize and deal with are the *non*-life-threatening situations that can throw your body and mind out of harmony. To get you started, complete this simple activity to figure out the types of stress that you are exposed to on a typical day.

POSSIBLE FIGHT-OR-FLIGHT TRIGGERS

Events	Time Spent (hours/minutes)
Traffic jam	
Crowded environment	
Work-related stress	
School-related stress	
Home-related stress	
Cell phone use	
Video streaming/TV watching	
Total	

The purpose of this exercise is to help you become more aware of how often you could be exposing yourself to false triggers of the fight-or-flight response. Say you have an eight-hour workday that is stressful already. After work, you are frequently checking your phone because of the urge to respond to non-urgent messages immediately. You intersperse "social media breaks" throughout the day to ensure that you are not missing out on anything fun. What ends up happening is that you are inviting mental stress for your body.

A person's health is hugely dependent on the unobstructed flow of Qi and blood within the body. Our emotions have a key role in shielding our ability to maintain dynamic balance. *Emotions that are not properly managed will be reflected in a person's performance or interactions with others.* For athletes, it is important to manage common stressors—things related to everyday training, competition for playing time, pressure leading up to games, or even false fight-or-flight triggers, which we will discuss in the next section—that might get overblown in the head. Emotions that are not properly managed will be reflected in an athlete's performance.

Start Simple

This is not a book about sports psychology, though interest in that discipline is growing rapidly. But we want to give you enough information to get you started down the path of paying attention to your emotions, how they are affecting your body, and how changes in your body might be reflected in your emotions.

Start by being mindful of your emotions. Let's be clear, mindfulness doesn't mean a ten-day retreat or a dedicated meditation space (although both would be beneficial). It means that you are more aware of what is happening around and inside you—having a deeper understanding of the real situation that you are in. Take some time to reflect on the types and duration of stimuli that you are exposing yourself to, and understand that at times you might be tricking your mind into a fight-or-flight response by activating your survival instincts.

You can also take steps to start minimizing the false fight-or-flight responses triggered in your body. Remember Bryan (one of Andy's clients) from the Introduction? Bryan had gone through a remarkable transformation after months of living in the extreme. But as soon as life threw him a curveball (as life tends to), everything was wrecked. He was looking to start a new business, which is already enormously stressful. On top of that, Bryan was always on Facebook and text messaging with friends: His in-person conversations with Andy were often about people's political comments on Facebook (which definitely stirred up his fight-or-flight system), and he would *always* reply to texts from Andy within five minutes.

To achieve his health and fitness goals, Bryan first needed to decrease the amount of false fight-or-flight triggers in his life. Instead of just instructing him to decrease time spent on social media and shallow phone conversations (because telling people to decrease social media time is equivalent to telling someone to quit smoking—it's not easy), Andy challenged Bryan to read two physical books (not e-books on a tablet or phone because of potential distractions). Andy's hope was that reading books would decrease the time Bryan spent on meaningless, shallow activities, and he would have more time to reflect on what he had read and on the different emotions he was encountering. Bryan also visited a massage therapist who followed the principles of TCM meridians. Since then, although he is not the skinny, transformed Bryan anymore, his weight is under control, and he is more aware of his emotions.

Analyzing Diet Is NOT Enough

The same concept of emotional balance applies to Ben from our case study. If we get too caught up in analyzing his diet, we will overlook an important aspect—emotion. Ben scored quite low on the Qi Stagnation section of the body constitution questionnaire, which suggests that he wasn't struggling with emotional problems. But looking at the nature of his job, it might also be possible that stress was affecting his digestion. After all, he is an investment banker, which is a mentally taxing job. For Ben to gain a comprehensive understanding of why he was experiencing poor digestion, he needed to not only examine his diet but also evaluate the amount of stress that he was exposing himself to. He would then need to be more mindful of how he reacted to different situations. As a result, he could get a more complete picture of the root cause of imbalance in his life.

ASSESS THE HEALTH OF YOUR FASCIA

The concept of healthy fascia is very similar to the concept of dynamic balance. A balanced and harmonious tension along the fascial meridians helps support fluid and silky movement. Too much or too little tension along the lines or bands of fascia can lead to muscle tension, movement deficiencies, poor posture, and ultimately pain.

In this chapter, we'll talk about three common causes of unhealthy fascia, as shown here:

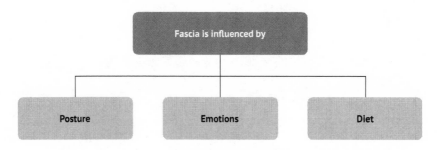

Factors influencing fascial health

Posture

To understand the effects of posture on fascia, we have to first remember that fascia adapts to the moves you make. Sometimes, the thickening of fascia helps to support the activities of daily life; other times, it may hinder our movement.

Your fascia will adapt to the position that it is frequently put to. Imagine the fascial meridians as rubber bands that are supposed to pull in different directions. In real life situations, different bands will pull in different directions depending on the movement that you do. The more you train yourself in certain positions, the more the fascia will continue to adjust. And that's the beauty of human movement—fascia is highly adaptable.

Think of Beyoncé when she is performing precise and emotionally charged dance moves on stage, Serena Williams winning matches with her thunderous serves, Michael Jordan dunking a basketball from the free throw line, or Tiger Woods and other golfers hitting crisp and penetrating shots that result in a hole in one. These athletes have trained for years and decades, and their fascia have adapted to their specific needs. The same is true for your body.

In the rest of this section, we'll look at some myths about posture and fascia and explain how you can do a better job of keeping all of your "rubber bands" healthy.

IS SITTING BAD OR GOOD?

The point about adapting to our lifestyles is best illustrated with an everyday example. Let us talk about sitting—sitting in a chair, to be precise. Most of us have a slightly slouched posture when sitting, as shown here:

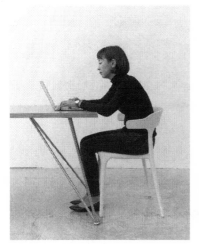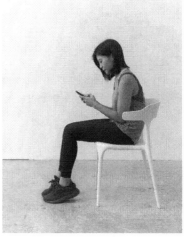

Sitting postures

In fact, the modern lifestyle demands that people sit in chairs more than ever before. We are always in this slightly hunched-forward position, whether in school, at work, or commuting between places. You have probably heard that sitting is the new smoking. While there is a degree of truth to this statement, *sitting is actually not inherently bad—but prolonged sitting is.*

You see, throughout human history, humans had to sit on rocks, trees, grass, and mud—whatever surface was available! Nowadays, "progress" has meant many of us sit in the same chair in the same position for hours at a time, day after day. Outside of work or school, we do not even need to physically go to the mall or the grocery store, as everything is accessible with the click of a button. Comedian Ronny Chieng once sarcastically joked in his Netflix comedy series that Amazon shipping is still too slow: "When I press buy, put the item in my hand, NOW!" Jokes aside, the cold hard truth is that this age of convenience usually leads to less movement for our bodies, and that, in turn, can lead to fasciae that are better suited for sitting than for the movement required of an athlete.

New York Times and *Wall Street Journal* bestselling author and physical therapist Kelly Starrett highlights the menacing consequences of prolonged sitting in *Deskbound*, a book he co-authored—namely that our shoulders, chest, and neck muscles become adaptively shortened and stiff. That is, we slouch. In a typical slouching position, the hips and the spine are flexed; the shoulders are protracted, elevated, flexed, and internally rotated; and the head protrudes forward. Over time, we are essentially initiating a performance-deflating loop where the lack of movement creates adaptive stiffness, stiffness compromises our ability to move, and our inability to move reinforces adaptive stiffness.

Could You Be a Queen's Guard?

To illustrate that *any* position can become harmful if you do it long enough, we want to challenge you to see how you'd perform as one of the royal guards at Buckingham Palace in London. These guards are renowned for rarely deviating from their stony expression and upright "perfect" posture, even when tourists are trying to provoke a reaction. Try this activity at home or at the gym: Have a stopwatch ready, and set it to a relatively short time, say twenty minutes. If there is enough space in your camera, set up a time-lapse recording to document your posture throughout the twenty minutes. The goal is to demonstrate perfect posture, as the Queen's Guard would, while doing whatever you would normally do (working, reading, writing, watching television). You don't have to stand like the Queen's Guard—you can be sitting—but the key is to maintain a perfect posture for your selected time period. Take note of your thoughts during this activity. What you should feel is that maintaining "perfect" posture for an extended period will also stiffen your body up. Our bodies are designed to move, not be still like a statue. The Queen's Guard experience should point to the first part of the overarching TCM principle: There is bad (body stiffens) in good (the "perfect" posture).

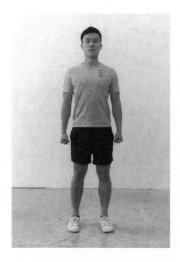

Queen's Guard posture

MY 20-MINUTE QUEEN'S GUARD EXPERIENCE

_____

_____

_____

_____

_____

How did it feel? Difficult to maintain? If you compare the Queen's Guard to our normal slouching posture, you might find that, surprisingly, the body will feel stiff _regardless_ of the posture that you are in. Once again, it's not so much the posture that is causing problems but the duration for which a posture is sustained.

Your fascia is designed to express different shapes and movements. Being stationary will stiffen your fascia and cause dehydration.

IS SLOUCHING ALL BAD?

Now that we've shown that neither sitting nor standing is inherently good if we do either one all the time, what about slouching? The hunched-over position of the slouch is being hammered by different health and fitness professionals, usually for the right reasons related to our preceding message: If you slouch all the time, that position is what your muscles and fascia will adapt to.

One of the first things that they teach you at a public-speaking class, or interview class, is to display an open posture—no slouching, hands out of pockets, and no crossed arms—to communicate openness or interest. The slouching posture is associated with feelings such as insecurity, anxiety, and boredom. Certainly, there cannot be goodness in this position?

Professor Go Igarashi and colleagues from Nagoya University in Japan once did a small study on the relationship between tasks that require a lot of thinking (cognitive tasks) and seating posture. They had twenty-eight Japanese fourth graders seated on backless stools and fitted with electrodes that tracked the activity level of their back muscles. To begin the study, the students were asked to sit in the upright position. Then they were separated into two groups. Half the group were told to sit quietly for two minutes, while the other half had to verbally answer math questions. The math questions started easy, then got increasingly difficult. The hardest questions were above their grade level. Interestingly, as the questions became more challenging, the students slouched more. The authors raised the question of whether tasks that require a lot of brain power may cause slouching posture because the brain is too busy thinking to worry about maintaining a "correct" posture.

Take a moment to think about the last time you solved a complex problem when you were at school or work: You were probably so laser focused on the problem at hand that you inadvertently slipped into a slouched position.

Going back to the book *Deskbound*, Kelly Starrett comments that sitting on chairs switches off our glutes, which means that we are using just our muscles in the trunk to keep our spine supported in its natural shape. Thus, maintaining an erect spine when sitting is a cognitively demanding task. And while many people think they are good at multi-tasking, the reality is that your brain doesn't really juggle multiple tasks well. If faced with two different tasks—sitting in a good posture and solving complex problems—your brain will direct more power for the problem at work or school.

In a way, then, the fact that the fourth graders ended up slouching meant that they were working hard!

Now, does this mean that slouching is good for you? Not really.

But slouching is not *all* terrible. There are times when slouching elicits something positive, such as freeing up cognitive space. And this brings us to the second part of the overarching TCM principle: There is a degree of good in bad.

Put those two parts together, and we get this—*There is a degree of bad in good, and there is a degree of good in bad*. Remember in the Yin-Yang sign that there is a dot of white in black and a dot of black in white? Good posture, a posture where joints are in *neutral* positions, has been promoted as the best and most ideal for the body, for logical reasons. But if you stand there all day like the royal guards at Buckingham Palace, you will also feel rigid and tight. The same can be said about bad posture. Slouching the entire day is detrimental to your physical and emotional health. But if you are working on a complex problem, it is normal to slouch a little bit.

Therefore, our view on poor posture is simple: *The only bad posture is prolonged idleness* (sitting in a chair for eight hours a day or standing at a desk for eight hours a day). Our bodies and fascial network are designed to have the tensile strength and fluidity to move into different shapes. Sure, there are optimal and biomechanically efficient postures that allow us to lift heavy things off the ground or to carry heavy loads around. But the truth is, it is not certain positions that make a posture bad; it is the prolonged and persistent duration that can cause problems such as dehydration. The body is designed to move and should be moved.

WHAT'S BAD? OVERUSE OR UNDERUSE

The performance-deflating loop we mentioned previously is known to the National Academy of Sports Medicine as the cumulative injury cycle. The cycle is described as cumulative because the injury might not have resulted immediately as the result of a single traumatic event (spraining an ankle from a jump landing, for example) but rather from repeated, more minor stresses.

Essentially, the cycle begins when the body begins to treat consistently shortened or lengthened muscles as dysfunctional tissue, which have poor circulation and are sticky and full of friction. You might even feel some knots when you touch a muscle in this condition, because the fascia has become rigid or "adhesive"—serving to hold the muscle fibers in one particular position rather than help the fibers glide over one another. These fascial adhesions are formed as a result of poor circulation and either too much or too little tension.

As the cycle continues, the impact is cumulative (gets worse), making injuries more frequent or worse than they otherwise would have been. Fascial adhesions compromise how muscles and their fascia move during a movement, which reinforces any overuse or underuse of these tissues that is already occurring. By knowing this cycle, athletes can understand the insidious nature of the tissue dysfunction and apply strategies to reverse the cycle by making sure that each muscle fascia gets regular use.

You can think of the cumulative injury cycle as a label for any consistent overuse or underuse of a muscle and its fascia. Overuse is at one end of the spectrum; lack of physical activity is at the opposite end. Your body and fascia do not like extremes. Too much or too little activity causes deviation from your dynamic balance.

The nature of the performance-deflating loop, or cumulative injury cycle, is best illustrated by an athlete.

Take a golfer, for example: Golf is a sport that requires repetitive swings from the right side to the left side for a right-handed golfer (left to right for left-handed golfers). A fluid and powerful swing like Tiger Woods's at the peak of his career demands tremendous mobility from the ankles, hips, spine, and shoulders. If a golfer sits at a desk in front of a computer for eight hours a day, chances are their hips and spine will tighten up from the lack of movement. The body will have adapted to this new restricted position, which means their ability to freely rotate will have diminished by the time the golfer starts hitting balls at the driving range. Like many golfers, rather than taking the time to loosen up, they are likely to continue hitting balls with restricted movement. Imagine doing a hundred swings during practice with restricted hips and back, then another hundred the day after, and so on. Basically, the golfer is creating a new movement pattern for the body. Not only are they not reaching their full potential, but they also are exposing themself to the risk of injury by practicing the restricted movements.

The Source and Cause of Pain

When it comes to pain, it is important to decipher whether the *source* of pain is the *cause* of the pain. Continuing the golfer example, let's look at a common golf injury: lower back pain. It accounts for about 25% of all golf injuries, so it's always good to understand and prevent it. If a golfer is experiencing lower back pain, the original cause is unlikely to be from a "weak lower back."

continued

In Chapter 1.4, we introduced the tensegrity model as a demonstration for healthy fascia. One of the points that we highlighted was the interconnective nature of the tensegrity model. That is, a compression or decompression in one area can cause tension at another. If we apply that to golf and lower back pain, a fluid golf swing demands tremendous mobility from the ankles, hips, spine, and shoulders. Since your muscles and fascia are all designed to move together to facilitate the most efficient energy transfer, if any of those joints have suboptimal range of motion, the lower back may be forced to produce rotational force (which isn't something that the lower back is oriented to do). At some point, forces accumulate (cumulative injury cycle), and the lower back gives up.

When looking at pain and discomfort, instead of hyper-focusing on the joint with the pain or discomfort, evaluate the mobility and movement pattern of surrounding areas.

Diet

We spent a lot of time discussing diet in Chapter 2.3 and won't review all the details here. But what you need to know is that one of the main benefits of having a balanced diet is so you can maintain healthy, elastic fascia. And that means paying attention to the types and amount of fluids and food that you consume.

TOO LITTLE WATER (DEHYDRATION)

Dehydration is one of the most common contributors to unhealthy fascia. Put simply, if the fascia is retaining less water, elasticity decreases. As renowned fascia researcher Robert Schleip points out in the book *Fascia in Sport and Movement*, water plays a critical role in lubricating fascia and muscle tissue. A lack of hydration means that instead of fascial layers sliding over one another without friction, different layers become gluey and sticky. Instead of gliding over each other like frictionless plastic, the fascia acts like Velcro trying to slide past each other. Yikes.

UNHEALTHY EATING

You are what you eat. What you put into your body has an energetic effect. If your ability to produce quality movements is heavily influenced by hydration, then it is only logical to assume that foods that dehydrate you will cause you more harm than good. With that said, you will not be able to find foods that directly lead to unhealthy fascia.

Emotions

To understand how posture—meaning the position of our muscles and fascia—affects our mood and performance, let's recall some of the concepts mentioned earlier about Yin-Yang. Recall how the back side of our body is referred to as Yang (and the front side Yin) because of the sunlight it receives while being on all fours.

General depression and anxiety are considered to be manifestations of excessive Yin suppressing the Yang's activity. (Sometimes it can also be comorbid with a lack of Yang, but that usually happens more in the elderly.) Therefore, those suffering this imbalance often give out a downward energy force where the body posture tends to lean toward the Yin side of the body, stretching out the back (the Yang surface) as a shield to protect themselves. Just like in boxing, when you anticipate a hit, you lean in, tuck your shoulders in, and have your belly tightened to minimize the damage you'll receive. Once the hit is done, you open back up and prepare to fight back. However, when it comes to depression and anxiety, there are no visible "enemies" for us to throw a punch at, leaving us in the protective mode.

THE DEADLY COMBO: PROLONGED SLOUCHING AND STRESS

Your fascia has a bigger role than helping you move.

In Chapter 1.4, we touched on how fascia senses emotion through a process called interoception. Interoception is a sense that helps us understand and feel what is going on inside the body. Through this sense we feel our heartbeat, respiration, and satiety, as well as the nervous system that pertains to emotions. In other words, interoception is the process that tells you whether you are maintaining dynamic balance. Sensory receptors for interoception are found beneath the skin and in the muscle and fascial tissues. Since fasciae permeate throughout the entire body, interoceptors are therefore located throughout the body.

Sensations That Fascia Helps Communicate

According to Robert Schleip, these sensations include warmth, coolness, pain, tickles, hunger, thirst, sexual arousal, muscular activity, heartbeat, distension of bladder, distension of stomach, and sensual touch.

We spent some time in the previous section talking about the insidious nature of prolonged idleness, namely prolonged sitting in modern society. Because sitting stiffens many muscles and fascia that should be moving, it elicits negative mental effects through interoception.

The link between posture and emotion is not a new concept. Professors John Riskind and Carolyn Gotay published a study in 1982 that suggests physical postures can affect emotional experience and behavior: "Subjects who were placed in a hunched, threatened physical posture verbally reported self-perceptions of greater stress than subjects who were placed in a relaxed position."[3] Notice that the word *threatened* was used to describe the hunched posture. We took photos of ourselves, shown next, to illustrate how posture and emotions are often connected.

---

3   Riskind, J. H. and C. C. Gotay. 1982. "Physical Posture: Could It Have Regulatory or Feedback Effects on Motivation and Emotion?" *Motivation and Emotion*, 6(3), 273–298. doi:10.1007/bf00992249.

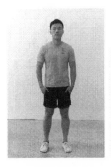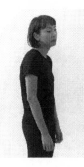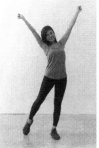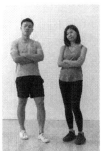

Posture and emotions

Slouching posture, from an emotional point of view, elicits negative emotions. Now we know why: The interoceptors will tell the brain that something is wrong and that the body needs to go into protective mode just in case it has to fight or flee. Starrett writes in *Deskbound* that slouching even tricks your mind into a fight-or-flight state by altering breathing mechanics. So when you slouch for a long time finishing that paper, binging on the latest Netflix series, or scrolling through Instagram from one post to the other, you are chronically challenging your body's ability to maintain dynamic balance.

FASCIA DURING FIGHT-OR-FLIGHT SITUATIONS

Our central nervous system receives the greatest amount of sensory input from the myofascial tissues (the fascia surrounding the muscles). In Chapter 2.4 on emotions, we talked about how a basic level of anxiety is needed to protect us from danger and to allow us to react faster to emergencies. However, inordinate amounts of anxiety are detrimental to one's performance. When faced with a stressor—emotional or physical—our bodies tense up so that we can fight it or flee from it.

Unfortunately, in a modern world filled with distractions, the list of stressors is forever growing, yet the majority are non-life-threatening. In addition to being stuck in traffic and scrolling through social media, we can add slouching to that list. (Check people's posture when they are angrily honking or swiping to check for the number of "likes" they have. More often than not, they are slouching! There we have another vicious cycle.)

Evaluating Fascial Health

The TCM concept of balanced health is predicated on the idea of smooth and unobstructed Qi and blood circulation throughout the body. A key area that must be considered is the fascial system. In this chapter, we identified three factors that influence the health of the fascial system: posture, diet, and emotions.

We talked about the Yin-Yang of posture, but not in the conventional understanding that certain postures are bad. A posture is truly detrimental if we are stuck in it for an extended period, like when we work or study, regardless of whether that posture is slouching or perfectly upright just like the royal guards at Buckingham Palace.

We then talked briefly about the cumulative injury cycle where unhealthy fascia deflates performance by limiting a muscle's or a joint's movement capabilities, which will reinforce that dysfunctional area. This is a common risk factor to all athletes. After all, sports practice is all about mastering a craft through repetition (a lot of Yang). Over time, overuse injuries may result.

The other two factors that may impact fascial health are diet and emotions, which relate to the previous chapters. Because fascia is mostly made up of water, hydration and dietary habits will have a direct impact. Fascia also plays a pivotal role in sensing the current state of health. If we choose to sit for eight hours a day, we might trick the system to be on fight-or-flight mode (Yang) by being rigid, tight, and having shallow breaths (qualities of the fight-or-flight response).

In short, our fascia is constantly being put under stress, and it's easy to create fascia that is stiff and clumpy versus elastic and slippery. Since we can't avoid all of the forces that push us toward imbalance, we have to be more deliberate about the keyword we introduced at the very beginning of this book: *recovery*. All the sweat, blood, and tears that you put in during practice to perfect your skill (Yang) must be counterbalanced by adequate recovery (Yin). Our goal is to reverse the cumulative injury cycle by understanding the root cause of imbalance, which may be that you are sitting too much or swinging a golf club too much without thinking about alleviating those overused muscles. Ultimately, we are looking for smooth, silky, and healthy fascia that allows your body to dance like Beyoncé, serve like Serena Williams, shoot a game-winning fadeaway shot like Michael Jordan, or swing the club like Tiger Woods.

How Healthy Is Your Fascia?

In Chapter 4.4, we provide a worksheet that you can use to evaluate your own fascia, so you can identify specific ways to create more balance.

Analysis of Ben's Fascia

To conclude this chapter, let's go back to the Ben case study one more time. Ben, as you may recall, was training to become bigger, faster, and stronger. But after three months of hard-core training, he was feeling sluggish and bloated, though he had gained muscle mass. On the surface, gaining mass seems to be a plausible cause of Ben's sluggishness. Should we then draw the conclusion that gaining mass is the root cause of his imbalance? Of course not! We have already looked at his diet (p. 100) and emotions (p. 117)—what can we now learn from an analysis of his activity (and the impact on his fascia)?

A couple of warning signs jumped out immediately:

- First, Ben has an office job, which means that he is exposed
  to prolonged idleness. Adding in his commute before and after
  work, which comes to a little more than an hour, he is stuck
  in the same seated posture for nine hours a day (not counting
  a few bathroom breaks and a lunch break to get some needed
  movement).

- Second, we gathered from his background story that he drinks a
  lot of coffee, which dehydrates the body.

- Third, he has a stressful job.

When added up, these factors create a classic deadly combo. Ben is
pretty much flooding his brain with a number of false fight-or-flight
triggering activities. It is not surprising that Ben is feeling sluggish and
lethargic, because his lifestyle invites imbalance (too much Yang, as
reflected in his constitution), which is killing his performance.

Knowing the connection and link among the three factors of diet,
emotions, and fascia, the question is, what strategies can Ben incorporate into his recovery routine so that his body can maintain dynamic
balance by alleviating and minimizing all the unnecessary Yang in his
life? We'll talk about ideas he can use in Part 3.

DEALING WITH IMBALANCES

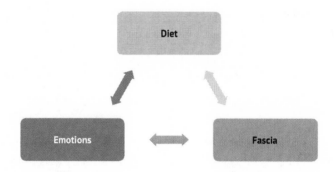

The purpose of this section was to show how the TCM concepts introduced in Part 1 can help you start identifying potential causes of imbalance, especially those linked to your diet, emotions, and fascia. Maintaining balance in these three areas is one way to help Qi and blood flow through your body; if the Qi-blood is blocked, too slow, or too fast, your athletic performance will diminish.

That's why, if you go to a TCM clinic, one of the first things that they will look at is your dietary habits. You are what you eat. Chapter 2.3 described how we must all eat according to our constitution, geographical location, and season. Eating foods outside of what is deemed natural is preposterous to firm TCM followers, as that implies a person is going against the law of nature.

With that said, however—and as important as dietary habits are—a strict and healthy diet could be overshadowed by negative emotions associated with stress. Consider a person that eats a double cheeseburger and fries, drinks a full-sugar soda, and tops that off with a chocolate donut every meal. While we would all agree that such a diet would eventually kill that person, if they are living a low-stress life, they will be far happier and healthier than someone who strictly follows the "perfect" diet but is stressed all the time about everything.

More generally, TCM frequently talks of the seven emotions and their interplay with different Zang-Fu organs. Dealing with emotions is a matter of management, not avoidance. We even applied the Yin-Yang philosophy to illustrate that while there are emotions that are generally positive, positive emotions will also have an element of negativity if not managed properly. The same can be said about negative emotions. Problems arise when emotions are heavily tilted toward one side of the spectrum.

Similarly, with fascia and movement, there are those on one end of the spectrum who do not move around much during the day, and at the other end are those who move too much, resulting in an overuse injury. Fascia also has an emotional side to it through the process called interoception. We also know that different postures might elicit different emotions. Someone who sits or stands in a slouched position might be applying all their cognitive power to finish a demanding task. Slouching is not inherently bad, but the mind will remain in the fight-or-flight state if the person continues to sustain that closed posture.

A Case Study of Imbalance vs. Dynamic Balance

To see how all of these factors come together when understanding imbalances, let's look at the story of Elise, one of co-author Stella's former clients. Elise worked hard at her office job, had recently separated from her partner, and was putting in a lot of time at the gym—to the point of developing the "Instagram-able" abs that people envy. However, she had one little secret that bothered her a lot. Her discharges were brownish, sticky, and often had an unpleasant smell. She visited multiple Western doctors, but nothing changed—except her menstruation cramps got more and more painful, to a point where it affected her work performance. This made her even more stressed and frustrated.

The first time Elise visited Stella, her body was very tense. Elise was a very nervous and anxious person. You could feel it by how fast she talked and the fact that she seemed to be always in a hurry—she wouldn't even stop to say "hi" to the nurses in Stella's clinic.

Elise's abs had the contours that athletes envy—but they were stiff. When Stella pressed down onto Elise's abs, it hurt. Stella could feel the lumps of knots all tangled together, and she suspected these knots were related to the constant accumulation of stress at work and the gym. When Elise became more static and less dynamic in her posture, the organs living inside her abdomen had to adapt to the new "fixed" environment of her hunched position. The discharges and smells were signs of the lack of fluidity in her muscles and how that was squeezing her internal organs and thus causing them to change. It's those micro-physical changes in the body that we don't realize have been gradually building up that cause the later structural and chemical changes.

Something about Elise's lifestyle was obviously out of balance. The stress from work, the high demands she set for herself, and the avoidance of the heartbreaking feelings from her breakup together caused a stagnation in the flow of her Qi. After a long period under this condition, the stagnated Qi had affected her body, and it manifested on the organs in the pelvis. The abnormal discharge was a sign that the Qi had affected the flow of the blood and other fluids in the body.

For Elise, the plan was to restore the balance, in both her life and her body, by focusing on the three elements discussed in this part of the book: fascia, diet, and emotions.

First, in terms of fascia, Elise needed to re-create space in her abs using the following:

- Active movements such as stretching and elongating the abdominal muscles

- Passive movements such as cupping and acupuncture to release tension, untangle the knots in the body, and free more space inside for the organs

Second, Elise needed to modify her dietary habits. Though it might have sounded as though she was eating healthily, her diet was out of balance with her constitution and nature. Her original diet consisted of mostly cold and raw food, turning her gut into something akin to a cold, wet, and slimy cave that occasionally drips water from the ceiling! What Elise needed to do was replace some of the foods that were cold in nature with foods warm in nature but not too nutritious. She made the following changes:

- She eliminated protein powder from her diet. Protein powder acts like dynamite in the body. Yes, dynamite is warm—but it explodes! What Elise needed instead was to slow down the pace of her body.

- She reduced the amount of cold and raw food like salads—as cold and raw foods are taxing for the digestive organ (following the TCM concept of organs)—and replaced them with cooked food or foods that are warm in nature, like ginger, rice, pumpkin, and onions. Elise was introducing these less-processed foods to help her digestive organs work better and spend less time and energy solving digestion puzzles. Note that certain cooking methods (e.g., baking and frying) can make foods that are cold and wet in nature warmer in nature.

Third, in terms of mood, Elise's anxiety and insecurity were the roots of her behavior. She needed to understand that sometimes if we want to achieve "peak" performance, we first need to embrace the "bottom" performances. Everything is dynamically changing. The only thing that remains still and constant is a dead object. It is normal to have different reactions to different stimuli in our environment, either feeling happy on a sunny day or gloomy on a rainy day. No state is ever constant; therefore, what we must learn to bring out our better performance is to adapt. When something we cannot control happens, we can more easily maintain dynamic balance if we focus on what we *can* control: diet, routines, and habits.

The journey for Elise was not easy. She had to build whole new habits very different from her previous ones. After six months of training and practice and revision on her movements and diets, her weight did not change much. But her abs were not as stiff as before. The discharges gradually went back to normal, and the bad smell disappeared. Her menstrual flow also improved, with fewer clumps of blood clots and only occasional and bearable cramps.

The stagnant backwater that was once Elise's body is now again a flowing stream. She still gets anxious at times, but at least now she takes the time to stop, take a break, and say "hi" to the nurses.

Look for Connections

One last reminder: Though we talked about each of the three main sources of imbalance—diet, emotions, and fascia—as neatly divided topics, don't forget that dynamic balance is ultimately about how everything is inseparably linked. Diet affects emotions, emotions affect fascia, and fascia can affect how you feel and your dietary needs. The connections between food, emotions, and fascia determine the body's basic physical and mental health. Understanding the interplay of each of the pairings will help you or your athlete untangle the imbalances that you are facing.

PART 3

LIFESTYLE STRATEGIES FOR DYNAMIC BALANCE: SOME PRACTICAL POINTERS

MANAGING DYNAMIC BALANCE IN THE BODY

The body is constantly trying to regulate its internal environment to maintain dynamic balance. Blockages, deficiencies, or even excessive amounts of Qi would compromise recovery quality and overall health. In this part, we will review a few techniques to help us better manage our bodies, including the following:

- Chapter 3.1: Developing a Diet for Optimum Health and Performance (suited to your constitution, the season, and geographical location)
- Chapter 3.2: Mastering the Art of Breathing
- Chapter 3.3: Developing Harmony in Your Movement
- Chapter 3.4: Incorporating TCM Recovery Tools

DEVELOPING A DIET FOR OPTIMAL HEALTH AND PERFORMANCE

As we mentioned at the end of Part 2, if you visit a TCM practitioner, one of the first issues they will address is your diet and whether it is in tune with your body constitution and nature. The TCM dietary practice includes the adjustment of the five flavors, the nature of food (Yin-Yang/cold-hot), and the consideration of seasonal, geographical, climate, and individual factors such as body constitution.

In TCM there is no distinct difference between food and medicine, meaning that food may be all the medicine you need. TCM doesn't offer a one-size-fits-all plan either; instead, there are general guidelines that you can apply based on your constitution, the season, and the climate where you live.

In short, dietary plans must be individualized. Here are the steps to create an individualized plan—then we'll take a more in-depth look at each one:

1. Think of food as medicine intended to create optimal health.

2. Consider your body constitution and how that should influence the nature of the foods you choose.

3. Strive for harmony between the five flavors.

4. As much as possible, eat foods in season and in accordance with the climate.

5. Include a variety of fruits and vegetables (grown locally as much as possible).

6. Eat foods that are culturally acceptable in your area.

7. Stop eating once you are 70% full—the 70% principle.

8. Focus on dynamic balance.

1. Food as Medicine

One of the unique concepts of TCM is that food and medicine share the same source, are based on the same theories, and have the same uses. Food is considered more than just sustenance; *food contains therapeutic properties and is usually prescribed by TCM practitioners as the first line of treatment.* Shannon Wongvibulsin, MD, PhD, used an illustration similar to the one shown in the following figure in an article on nutrition. Her point was that TCM links "heat syndrome" (includes palpitations, a red face, anxiety, insomnia, constipation, and migraines/headaches) to stress and prescribes cooling foods to decrease the stress-induced "heat" and restore balance.

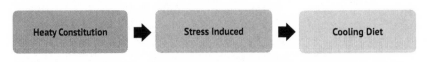

How to counteract "heat syndrome"

Compare that train of thought to the following figure, which summarizes the thinking we presented in Part 2. Look familiar?

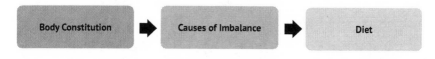

Body constitution and diet

In the following example, Wongvibulsin demonstrates how we should go about correcting imbalances if we suffer from heat syndrome:

1. Understand our current body constitution.

2. Consider where and how we developed the heat syndrome.

3. Develop a dietary strategy to combat the imbalance.

This three-step process can be applied to any situation where the body is out of balance. In every case, one of the first corrective strategies you should consider is changing what you eat. We acknowledge that it takes years of training and clinical practice before a TCM doctor can prescribe specific food and herbal remedies to an individual, but what we'll do in the rest of this chapter and elsewhere in the book is provide basic principles that you can apply to your own life.

2. Body Constitution and the Nature of Food

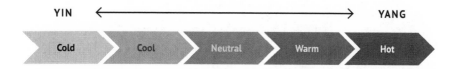

In the words of Harriet Beinfield and Efrem Korngold, authors of *Between Heaven and Earth: A Guide to Chinese Medicine*, "The appropriateness of a food cannot be established without knowledge of the context—not everyone will benefit equally from foods that contain the same measure of nutrients."[4]

---

4   Beinfield, H. and E. Korngold. 1991. *Between Heaven and Earth: A Guide to Chinese Medicine*. New York: Random House Publishing Group.

Every person has a unique constitution or body type that changes over time. Your constitution affects how you feel and behave. Therefore, a tailored dietary approach should be implemented to maintain your body's Yin-Yang. The criteria for selecting foods according to body constitution relate to balancing a person's Yin and Yang, as Beinfield and Korngold pointed out: "[People] who are cold and dry need warm, moisturizing food; people who are hot and damp need cool, drying food; people with congestion need decongesting food; and people who are depleted need replenishing food." As we learned in Chapter 2.1, sometimes it is difficult to classify a person into only one body constitution, as humans are complex and often fall into multiple constitution types. If that is the case for you, refer back to your body constitution questionnaire, list your predominant constitutions, and do your best to balance out the requirements of those differing constitutions.

Cooking Tips

Here are a few cooking tips that apply to us all, no matter our body constitution:

- Use fresh, organic, and seasonal foods.
- Cook food and serve it warm to help digestion.
- Steaming, poaching, and boiling help preserve the cool nature of food.
- Deep-frying, stir-frying, and roasting change the nature of food to be warmer.

The following table summarizes the key dietary guidance for each of the constitution types (you can find details about which foods to eat and which to avoid in Appendix D).

**SUMMARY OF DIETARY STRATEGIES ACCORDING
TO BODY CONSTITUTION**

Constitution	Strategy
Qi Deficiency	Eat foods that nourish the spleen and the gut.
Yang Deficiency	Eat foods that are neutral, warm, and nourishing.
Yin Deficiency	Eat foods to clear deficient heat. Avoid stimulating foods and drinks.
Phlegm-Wetness	Eat foods to nourish the spleen and to clear phlegm and dampness. Avoid raw, cold, oily, and heavily processed foods.
Wetness-Heat	Eat nourishing foods to clear deficient heat.
Qi Stagnation	Eat foods that stimulate Qi.
Blood Stasis	Eat foods that stimulate blood.
Balanced Health	No changes needed. Eat a variety of foods. Stay in balance!

3. Harmony of the Five Flavors

If you have jumped ahead to Part 4, you may have already completed a three-day food journal similar to the journal we showed for Ben in Chapter 2.3. If so, how did you fare? The goal of a balanced diet is to consume a variety of flavors, unless a certain flavor is contraindicative to your constitution. The Chinese believe that every bite of food sends the nutrients to the corresponding organ through the meridians:

- **Salty** (Kidney): Lubricates the intestines and helps remove waste accumulation

- **Sour** (Liver): Helps to control Qi, blood, and spirit; promotes digestion

- **Bitter** (Heart): Helps to dry dampness and calms the mind
- **Sweet** (Spleen): Tonifies (increases the available energy of) and moistens other herbs; lubricates dry conditions
- **Spicy** (Lung): Promotes Qi and blood circulation

Notice that we used the word *harmony* related to the five flavors instead of *balanced*. The danger of using the word *balance* is that people sometimes will interpret that as having to consume equal amounts of all flavors in their diet. This is not the case. In music, harmony is the composite product of individual musicians voicing together to form a cohesive whole. The goal of such practice is to produce music that is pleasing to the ear. In the same vein, harmony of the five flavors is achieved by collectively eating what is pleasing to the body. Depending on your individual factors (body constitution, the season, where you live), you may need to consume more bitter foods, or you might need to cut back on spicy foods, and so on.

Whole Grains Are Important!

If you go to any Chinese restaurant, you will be served rice along with other dishes. Rice is a type of whole grain, and grains are recognized as the foundation of human vitality. TCM considers grains to be beneficial to digestion by strengthening the stomach, small intestine, spleen, and pancreas. They are beneficial for all types of body constitutions.

The taste of grains is generally sweet, which tonifies the spleen and the stomach. Other grains include soybeans, wheat, broomcorn, millet, hemp, and beans. Eat a variety of whole grains that are grown locally and naturally. There is a concern about glutinous grains such as wheat, rye, and barley in modern nutrition. They are considered unsuitable for those who have a warm constitution, because glutinous grains are warming in nature.

4. Eat According to Season and Climate

It is six o'clock in the morning in the middle of a cold winter. The alarm clock goes off and you crack open the curtains, just to see that it is still dark outside. You struggle to get out of bed, give yourself the biggest pep talk, yet still struggle with motivation throughout the day. If you have experienced winter tiredness, don't worry, because you are not alone! Winter morning is a testing time for many people, and athletes are no exception. Humans are immensely influenced by changes in seasons and climates. We naturally want to sleep and rest during those cold winter days. On the other hand, if we wake up to a clear blue sky in the middle of July, the urge is to enjoy some sunshine outdoors.

Eating foods that are in season can alleviate the dampness, hotness, dryness, and coldness experienced in spring, summer, autumn, and winter. This is where the nature of foods comes into play, because of the effects that food elicits from the body. The ancient Chinese believed that seasonal foods naturally meet the nutritional needs of the area. Similar concepts can be found in other parts of the world.

Not too long ago, human diets consisted of what could be grown, foraged, or hunted throughout the year. In a globalized world, we can now go to the nearby grocery store to buy just about anything, no matter the season. But there is more to eating than convenience. The lure of convenience may interrupt the harmonic nature of your body, your performance, and your health. Stay away from the watermelons in the winter; save them for the next poolside party in the summer.

Bone Broths Once in a While

Bone broth has been around for centuries in Asian cultures. Recent research indicates that it is full of collagen, gelatin, glycine, glutamine, minerals, and electrolytes, which are great for soft tissue repair, digestive health, and immune function. Plus, it is a great dish for the winter season due to its warming nature, so cut back on the raw cold foods and have some bone broth instead.

5. Eat a Variety of Fruits and Vegetables Grown Locally

Imagine that there is an organic garden near you that grows various kinds of fruits and vegetables. Imagine walking into an orchard and handpicking some perfectly ripened apples. Now compare that with the apples grown in a mass production house, full of chemical fertilizers, then packaged and sold in a supermarket chain. Though the nutritional values of the apples might be similar, one is far more appealing than the other. TCM is all about living in harmony with the surrounding environment. Support local farms and eat foods that are grown locally as much as possible. Plus, purchasing fruits and vegetables from local farms will ensure that you are eating foods in season!

6. Eat Culturally Acceptable Foods

What foods are and are not culturally acceptable varies widely across the globe. Take horsemeat, for example. It has a darker appearance than beef, in part because it has twice the iron and almost the same amount of omega-3 fatty acids as farmed salmon. But the acceptance of horse-meat as a diet staple is championed in some parts of the globe and abhorred in others.

American journalist Caty Enders published an article in *The Guardian* about the decision in 2013 by a number of high-end restaurants to introduce horsemeat to the modern American palate. The result was disastrous. She wrote: "If you're like the majority of US citizens, you would likely balk—maybe even gag—at the thought of eating horsemeat at a restaurant. Horses are considered a delicacy in countries around the world, from Italy to China to Iceland, but Americans just can't seem to stomach the idea, even though many areas of arable public lands are currently overrun with about 50,000 feral horses—and bringing them to the dinner table might be one of the best possible solutions to the overcrowding."[5] The rest of the article went on to examine the reasons why Americans are reluctant to eat horsemeat.

Horsemeat is nutritious. But if eating horsemeat is culturally unacceptable, then stay away from it. The TCM philosophy calls for people to live in harmony with the surrounding environment. *If something is culturally unacceptable, it should be avoided.* The same idea can be applied toward the contentious topic of endangered species. Animal activists will criticize TCM practitioners over the use of endangered animals and species. As a response, we reiterate the words of Dr. Lixing Lao, a distinguished TCM scholar and practitioner whom we referenced in the Introduction. Lao has said that the use of endangered animals is indeed against the fundamental principle of TCM, where harmony between humans and nature must be maintained. Basically, there is always a substitute for the food or item that is not accessible.

7. 70% Principle

The 70% principle can be dated as far back as five hundred years ago, when TCM practitioners advocated for eating only to 70% of your capacity. Anything over the 70% mark will overwork the spleen and the stomach, impairing the organs' abilities to digest and nourish the body.

Think about typical North American meals, such as a sixteen-ounce New York strip from your local steakhouse, a chicken burrito from Chipotle, or two big pieces of Chicago-style pizza. While they are all delicious, most people have difficulty finishing the entire thing, especially if they have already consumed some appetizers that are equally huge in portion. By the end of the meal, most people are just so full that the meal is no longer enjoyable. And it certainly isn't nutritious.

---

5   Enders, C. 2015. "Why You Really Should (but Really Can't) Eat Horsemeat." January 9, 2015. Retrieved December 29, 2020, from https://www.theguardian.com/environment/2015/jan/09/eating-wild-horsemeat-america.

So, at your next mealtime, remember to eat until you are only 70% full (based on your own perception that you still have room for more). Have some water in between. Enjoy the meal. Pack the unfinished food and take it home for another meal at a different time.

8. Focus on Dynamic Balance

In Chapter 2.3, we outlined the differences in how the Chinese and Western languages describe the properties of food. Most strength and conditioning coaches are taught to evaluate foods based on carbohydrates, proteins, vitamins, minerals, calories, and other nutritional content. However, in the Chinese diet, the emphasis is not on macro- and micronutrients but rather the energetic properties of food. Each food has an associated nature, flavor, and Zang-Fu. The nature describes the therapeutic effects of the food on the body, while flavor describes the taste and the organ or organs associated with the food. Whether we describe food by the chemical reaction at the cellular level or by taste and energetic properties, we arrive at the same general conclusion: Every bite of food is not only giving you energy but also eliciting a chain of reactions from different body parts. At the end of the day, every natural food is nutritious.

Naomi Parrella, a medical doctor and an assistant professor at Rush University, wrote in a column published on the news website The Hill: "Even though there are multiple paths to being healthy and they may be different for each individual, to be sure, some healthy behaviors are more universal. This includes cutting back on sugar and processed foods and increasing daily physical activity and social connectedness contribute to everyone's well-being."[6]

In *The Yellow Emperor's Classic of Medicine*, the poetic phrase used to guide what we eat is to "use grains to nourish, fruit to assist, livestock

---

6　　Parrella, N. 2020. "Good-for-You Foods: One Size Does Not Fit All." The Hill. March 12, 2020. Retrieved December 28, 2020, from https://thehill.com/opinion/healthcare/487181-good-for-you-foods-one-size-does-not-fit-all.

to benefit, vegetables to supplement." The catch? They have to be of the right amount. So you should avoid excess intake of any one particular food. Check your body constitution and the season, and consume foods that belong to that season. Support a local farm and make friends with them. Developing an optimal diet is the critical first part of our strategy for achieving and maintaining dynamic balance. You'll find more instructions for developing your own dietary plan based on your constitution in Chapter 4.2, and you'll find reference material on foods and their nature and flavors in Appendix C.

MASTERING THE ART OF BREATHING

The second lifestyle strategy to work into your fitness plan is to improve your breathing. While breathing happens naturally every second of our lives, as an athlete you know that not all breathing is the same. What your lungs and core muscles have to do to maintain life is different from what they must do to drive peak performance. And that's why it's important to understand the mechanisms of breathing more fully and understand how to control and improve those mechanisms to maintain dynamic balance.

Breathing and Chinese Medicine

In Western anatomy, the lungs are part of the respiratory system. In TCM, the understanding of the lungs goes beyond their mechanical qualities: Qi comes not only from the food we eat but also from the air we breathe. Lungs in the TCM view are responsible for maintaining healthy immune defenses against pathogens, as well as circulating Qi and fluids throughout the body.

The lungs' paired Fu organ is the large intestine (see p. 62), whose main function is to release and eliminate undigestible material (stools). TCM further suggests that the large intestine relies on the following to perform its function:

- The downward movement of Qi executed by the lungs
- The moistening fluids pulled along with the downward Qi movement

Together, the lungs and large intestine build a defensive wall of Qi (also called Wei-Qi) so that the body will not be penetrated by outside pathogens. Any deficiencies in the lungs can affect the skin, sweat glands, and body temperature.

Since breathing is the first pathway for energy to enter our bodies, it is imperative that we pay attention to the quality of our breaths. Together with the food we eat, inhaled air is sent down to the spleen, where it is then transformed into the essence that supports our body's health. Poor breathing practices will impair the state of the lungs and the spleen, which will affect our energy level and immune system—a big red flag for any athlete.

THE DIAPHRAGM

Lung function relies to a great extent on the diaphragm, one of the most important muscles of the body. Continuously working to sustain life, the diaphragm is a huge dome-shaped muscle that is connected to the lower rib cage and the bottom of the spine. During inhalation, the diaphragm contracts by moving downward and widening. It is this contraction, with the assistance of the intercostals (muscles between the ribs), that pulls air into the lungs. During exhalation, the diaphragm and intercostals relax, which pushes air out of the lungs.

The diaphragm also has a second important role—to stabilize the central core of our body, which is why improving the breathing muscles and fascia should be a standard part of every athlete's workout, as we'll discuss later in this chapter.

UNDERSTANDING BREATHING MUSCLES

Though the diaphragm is the most critical breathing muscle, other muscles are involved as well. Normal breathing requires the use of primary breathing muscles, whereas heavy breathing requires assistance from secondary breathing muscles (see the following table). The action of normal resting breathing is typically called *belly breathing* because the abdominal region is heavily involved. As breathing becomes harder, it can be seen as *chest breathing* because the secondary muscles are recruited to help lift the rib cage, allowing the lungs to expand farther.

PRIMARY AND SECONDARY BREATHING MUSCLES

Primary Breathing Muscles	Secondary Breathing Muscles
Diaphragm Intercostals	Upper trapezius Scalenes Sternocleidomastoid Levator scapulae Pectoralis minor

Prolonged Shallow/Stress Breathing

You've probably had moments before an important game or competition where your heart is pounding, your muscles are tensing, and your breath is coming in short bursts. This type of breathing is called *shallow breathing*, and it can throw your body out of balance if you do it too long or too often (as is the case with the modern lifestyle). Deep breathing, in this case, does the opposite by restoring and maintaining balance. Let's look at each of these types of breathing.

Here we run into a chicken-and-egg situation like the performance-deflating loop in Chapter 2.5. Yes, shallow breathing can create imbalance, but anxiety, stress, and poor posture can lead to shallow breathing (creating what we call a performance-deflating loop). *Shallow* refers to how deeply you take air into your body. In shallow breathing, you take a small amount of air into the throat and upper chest area, as opposed to fully filling your lungs. So instead of expanding the lungs using the primary muscles first and the secondary muscles in support for a fuller breath, the accessory muscles get overworked, and the primary muscles underworked. In other words, the sequence has changed. Shallow breathing can trigger a fight-or-flight nervous system response, which, as we've discussed (p. 132), is used to prime the body for physical activity. Effectively, shallow breathing places the body in a state of heightened stress.

The following table compares the effects of belly/deep breathing and chest/shallow breathing. Breathing techniques can be used to induce a nervous system response from the body and are useful in different circumstances, as in you can actually use your breath to your advantage for different situations. For instance, you might need to calm down before that important free throw (belly/deep breathing) or prime yourself as you step up to bat after a long inning (chest/shallow breathing).

NORMAL VS. SHALLOW BREATHING

Normal Breathing	Shallow Breathing
Deep and long breaths	Shallow and short breaths
Belly breathing	Chest breathing
Calming	Priming
Activates relaxation response	Activates stress response

While shallow breathing can be used to prime the body prior to physical exertion, prolonged shallow breathing can be detrimental for the body and the mind in the long term. We have talked about the seven emotions and the danger of having one emotion dominating our life, and physically, compromised breathing could lead to tightness in the back, neck, and shoulders and the weakening of muscles in the core and pelvic floor.

The Mental Side of Breathing

We can prime the mind into fight-or-flight mode through short and shallow breathing, or we can do the opposite—calm the mind through slow and controlled diaphragmatic breathing. Since breathing directly controls the autonomic nervous system, focused lower belly breathing initiates the body's restoration process by initiating a rest-and-digest nervous system response, which lowers blood pressure and increases the overall oxygen level of blood; it also helps the brain register new movement patterns.

Breathing Should Be a Part of Your Core Workout

People usually associate core training with rock-hard and well-defined six-pack abs. While having a six-pack is cool and desirable—especially when you are on holiday at a beach resort—core training is much more than training the superficial layer of muscles that we see. There are different layers to the core.

While the outer layer of the core is most suitable for a beach show-off, it is the inner layers—such as the transverse abdominis—that do the work of assisting the diaphragm with breathing and stabilizing the spine. All of these qualities are critical to injury prevention, athletic performance enhancement, and overall postural stability.

Dr. Stuart McGill, a renowned expert in spinal health and back pain and professor at the University of Waterloo whose research revolves around back pain, coined the phrase "proximal stability for distal mobility" when it comes to core training. This phrase refers to the fact that athletes need to have a stable midsection or core (proximal stability) to maximize the range of motion in their extremities (distal mobility). That is, an athlete must have core stability for optimal extremity movements and function, and high-quality movements are not possible without a stable core. It follows that you should focus on training those stabilizing muscles that wrap around the spine, starting with the deepest layer. What are those muscles that form the core of the core? Your breathing muscles! Therefore, if you cannot breathe correctly, you cannot move correctly. Breathing training, or respiratory muscle training, must be part of your core training routine.

Progressive, Mindful Approach

With all the benefits associated with deep breathing, countless strength and conditioning coaches, wellness instructors, and therapists are instructing others to take deep diaphragmatic breaths.

But as with everything related to the TCM view, remember that our approach comes down to extremes versus finding balance. A progressive, flexible, and tailored approach is needed when working with different clients and athletes. The coach's role is to progressively introduce better breathing mechanics to their athletes' lives. Athletes don't have to suddenly be doing deep breaths *all the time*. Most just need to be more aware that they are stressed out. Remember, striving for dynamic balance is a process, not perfection.

Deep Breathing for Stress Reduction

In Chapter 4.5, we describe a very simple breathing exercise you can do to practice deep breathing. It's great for stress reduction, too. See p. 233 for instructions.

Improving Posture and Emotions

In Part 2, we discussed how posture and emotions are related. So one of the obvious ways you can improve the balance of your emotions is to get out of the vicious loop created by being in a slouching posture. Also, you can become more mindful of your breathing throughout the day and incorporate deep breathing as much as you can—and add deep breathing to your normal exercise routines.

If you study the science of breathing, you can quickly fall into a rabbit hole, as there are countless philosophies on the topic. For the purposes of our book, we'd like you to work on your breathing by emphasizing these three things:

1. Include respiratory muscle training, as those deep core stabilizing muscles are sometimes overlooked.

2. Use breathing training as a means to improve the lungs, which can improve overall immune functions.

3. Take a progressive and mindful approach to breathing.

When You Find Yourself Doing Shallow Breathing

1. Ask yourself whether the shallow breathing fits the situation. If yes, no further action is needed. If not, move to step 2.

2. Recognize that you are not in a life-threatening situation.

3. Try to breathe from your *belly.*

4. Inhale smoothly; make sure your body is in a position to provide unobstructed flow from your nose to your lungs.

5. Exhale fully.

6. Do not hold your breath!

7. Repeat the cycle a few times.

DEVELOPING HARMONY IN YOUR MOVEMENT

The demands of athletic movements require a sophisticated inter-action between the nervous system, the musculoskeletal system, and the connective tissues tied to different body parts. Therefore, good movement is not limited to isolated muscle strength but rather the harmony in which the different systems are operating. Take a basketball player, for example: To be a good rebounder of the basketball, the player must, of course, be able to jump well, but also have upper body strength to "box out" other players who are also trying to get the rebound. More important, they need to be able to produce all those movements at a precise moment, or they won't get the rebound.

That's why the third strategy for becoming better at dynamic balance is to improve the elasticity of your fascia by incorporating movement-based training. Movement is a great way to improve the overall health of the body. We purposefully stay away from the term *exercise* because many would associate that with running or gym workouts. We also assume that you exercise a fair amount since you are likely an athlete, so this chapter will present a routine that will add another dimension to your training. To kick it off, let's talk about fitness machines and isolated muscle work, a topic we've touched on before.

Are Isolation Machines Compromising Your Performance?

As we've discussed, traditional gym training focuses on building strength and mass one muscle group at a time. Rather than training the body as an interconnected unit, you are training different body parts in isolation. The problem with some traditional fitness equipment is that most of these machines do not require cohesive movements from different body parts. To quote physical therapist Gray Cook, one of the most influential minds in the fitness industry and the founder of Functional Movement Systems, from his book *Movement*:

> Modern fitness equipment allows training while sitting and even slouching comfortably. This equipment accommodates pushing and pulling with the arms, and flexing and pressing with the legs. The equipment also furnishes torso flexion, extension and rotation without forcing users to balance on their feet or naturally engage the stabilizing musculature.[7]

As the quote suggests, Cook is certainly not a fan of training only on isolation equipment, performing exercises. And he is absolutely spot-on: Since the body is one interconnected unit, you must learn to move different parts in an integrated manner.

Likewise, we have previously established that prolonged and repetitive postures—such as those produced in isolated muscle training—can also directly impact our fascia, our emotions, the flow of Qi-blood, and our ability to maintain dynamic balance. Isolated muscle training has

---

7   Cook, G. 2017. *Movement: Functional Movement Systems: Screening, Assessment and Corrective Strategies.* Santa Cruz, CA: On Target Publications.

its place, however. There are situations where training on a machine is useful and functional, such as during rehabilitation or hypertrophy phases. Rather than completely abandoning isolated muscle training, we can deliberately add in movement training that requires total body coordination, mobility, and stability.

Fascia Training

Because we now know about the connection between healthy fascia and overall health, training for healthier fascia should be a priority. Leading fascia researchers like Dr. Robert Schleip and Thomas Myers have long advocated for the idea of a fascia-oriented training approach. That is, instead of training muscles in isolation, we should include exercises that target different myofascial lines (groups of muscles), and exercises that improve or maintain the elasticity and sensory functions of fascia.

The idea of fascia training is not new. As Schleip and Divo Müller admit in their published journal article, "Training Principles for Fascial Connective Tissues: Scientific Foundation and Suggested Practical Applications," none of the typically recommended movements are completely new. In fact, as they point out, many aspects of known movement practices—like rhythmic gymnastics, modern dance, plyometrics, Gyrokinesis, chi running, yoga, or martial arts, just to name a few—"have been inspired by an intuitive search for elegance, pleasure and beauty, and/or they were often linked with non-fascia related theoretical explanation . . ." Turns out, humans have been practicing rhythmic movements that train the interconnected fascial system. We just did not have a scientific explanation for it until recently.

The goal of fascia training is to build an elastic and resilient body. As Schleip and Müller allude to in the same article, the intention of fascia-oriented training is to have a "more injury-resistant and resilient 'silk-like body suit,' which is not only strong but also allows for a smoothly gliding mobility over wide angular ranges." We provide examples of such training with our Five Animal Movements practice, which we'll review in the rest of this chapter.

Five Animal Movements Practice

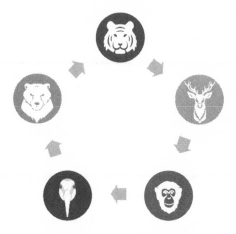

Animal-mimicking fitness routines have grown in popularity in recent years. The concept of imitating different animals has been around for millennia in China. For example, the "Five Animal Frolics" (*Wu-Qin-Xi* in Chinese) was created by physician Hua Tuo (circa 140–208 AD) some two thousand years ago. Hua Tuo is often referred to as the father of Chinese surgery and was one of the earliest advocates of Chinese sports medicine. He was best known for his surgical operations and the development of an anesthetic formula using herbs; meanwhile, he promoted regular exercises as a method of rehabilitation, recovery, and most important, sickness prevention. What a familiar message! Exercising improves Qi and blood circulation, which leads to better health and longevity.

The Five Animal Frolics is practiced by mimicking movement patterns of a tiger, deer, monkey, crane, and bear. Instructions on the movements were found in the book *Records of Nourishing the Body and Extending Life*, written around the sixth century. Different iterations and spinoffs have been created since the original, but no matter which variation you use, there are two main benefits to these integrated movements: They require adequate range of motion from different body parts (mobility) and the ability of your body to remain stable throughout the movements (stability).

BENEFIT 1: MOVING YOUR BODY THROUGH ALL PLANES OF MOTION

We live in a three-dimensional world, and our bodies are designed to move in different directions. Thus, there are three planes of motion:

1. **Sagittal** movements typically involve predominantly moving forward and backward.

2. **Frontal** movements typically go from side to side.

3. **Transverse** movements typically involve any form of twisting or rotation.

While daily human movements are mostly sagittal, the frontal and transverse planes must not be neglected. The following table indicates which planes of motion apply to each animal movement.

Tiger	Monkey	Bear	Crane	Deer
• Sagittal	• Sagittal • Transverse	• Frontal • Transverse	• Sagittal	• Frontal • Transverse

Planes of movement involved in the Five Animal Movements practice

BENEFIT 2: INCORPORATING QUADRUPEDAL MOVEMENTS

As you'll see, many of the Five Animal exercises involve quadrupedal movements (where your body is positioned with both hands and both knees on the ground, also known as being on all fours). Such movements are the foundation of efficient bipedal (where just both feet are on the ground) biomechanics. Recent research suggests that quadrupedal movements are beneficial in improving core stability (proximal stability), cognitive flexibility, and proprioception. Although most of our daily activities are bipedal, the use of quadrupedal movement patterns can improve coordination, control, and overall bipedal movement efficiency. After all, we all spent at least a few months on the floor crawling when we were babies! This is the time when babies discover that contralateral movements are the most efficient way to move—that is, if they move their *right* leg forward, they move their *left* arm next, then the left leg followed by the right arm. The opposing movement of the hips and shoulders provides both power and stability. Improving the quality of quadrupedal movements has a carryover effect to bipedal movements.

Quadrupedal movements also teach the body to move as an integrated unit. The body is a system of systems, and different systems must learn to produce movements in harmony rather than working in isolation. Moving well on all fours demands both stability and mobility from different joints and body parts. To move well, proximal stability around the mid-torso area is needed for mobility of distal joints such as the shoulders, hips, and ankles. Therefore, quadrupedal movements are also great core exercises, as trunk muscles are required and involuntarily "activated" during the movements.

The Five Animal Movements Routine

For the rest of this chapter, we'll give a brief overview of the Five Animal Movements series of exercises. We will also explore how a two-thousand-year-old fitness routine is validated by recent trends and findings in exercise science. The specific instructions for this routine are given in Chapter 4.6.

Speed of Movement

The speed of your movements should always be driven by intent. If you are using the routine as a warm-up, go at a faster tempo. If you are using the routine as part of a strength, endurance, or mobility workout, go slower. Fast is more Yang; slow is more Yin. Since our book is on recovery (Yin), we recommend that you go slowly. The sustained stretches during these movements will give your body a chance to calm down. And that can facilitate the kind of repatterning that addresses fascial adhesion and obstruction.

1. Tiger/Awareness

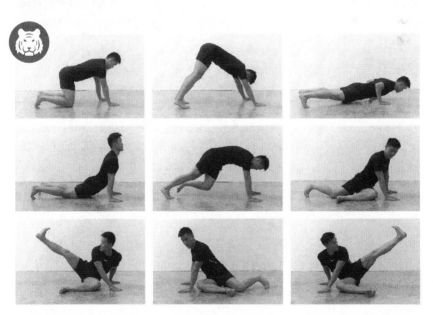

When a tiger hunts, it stretches and then compresses its spine as it takes enormous leaps while pursuing its dinner. But before engaging in such a demanding activity, what does a tiger do? Just like a house cat, it stretches its spine up and down to activate the muscles, nerves, and fascia—priming its body for action! We humans should do the same.

In the Tiger series of movements, you begin in a quadrupedal position (hands and knees on the ground) and move the hips and knees upward while the arms remain straight and hands are flat on the ground. Then you shift until your knees are back on the ground and your head and torso are upright. The purpose of this series of movements is to help you become more aware of the front and back sides of the body, and to activate the hip muscles in the second part of the series. While your head and torso are upright, you will lean to the left side and raise the right leg to mimic a tiger stretching its head. Then do the opposite side. This involves the meridians and fascial lines listed in the following table.

MERIDIANS AND FASCIAL LINES INVOLVED IN THE TIGER MOVEMENTS

Meridians	Fascial Lines
Spleen, stomach, liver, and kidney	Superficial and deep front lines
Bladder	Superficial back line

When performing the Tiger movements, pay attention to the rhythm of your movements—you are mimicking the elegance of a tiger in motion, not a stiff robot! During practice, there should be a smooth feeling to the movements.

BENEFITS OF THE TIGER MOVEMENT

The series of Tiger movements works great as an activation and integration drill, especially when you are stuck in front of a desk the entire day.

We say "activation" because you are engaging fascia and muscles along most of your body, lengthening the fascial back lines while shortening the front myofascial lines, then doing the reverse (shortening of the back lines and lengthening of the front lines). The first part of the exercise can be thought of as an integration drill because the movements require the interplay between the front and back fascial lines. The second part can be thought of as an activation drill of the hip muscles, which have been turned off and dehydrated from sitting all day.

2. Deer/Gracefulness

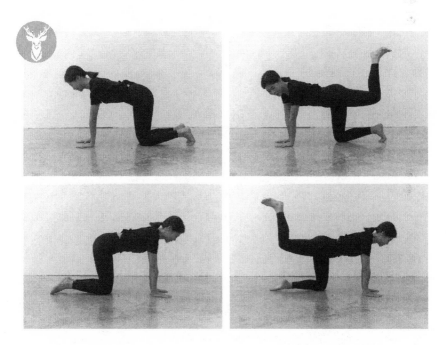

Deer have very graceful movements as they bound through the forest. They change the direction of their movement with the flick of a tail without missing a step. That requires strength and flexibility along the spine.

In the Deer movement, you once again begin in a quadrupedal position. Next, you raise and stretch one leg, then turn your head to look at the foot on that side—then repeat those steps on the other side. This bending of the spine from side to side helps improve mobility and involves the meridians and fascial lines listed in the following table.

MERIDIANS AND FASCIAL LINES INVOLVED IN THE DEER MOVEMENT

Meridians	Fascial Lines
Liver, gallbladder, small intestine, and triple burner	Lateral

BENEFITS OF THE DEER MOVEMENT

In recent years, the fitness industry has shifted its long-held notion on spinal mobility and stability. Athletes formerly were told to brace everything as they moved. However, the traditional notion that you want to have perfectly aligned movements has changed over the years. The industry now recognizes that the human body should have the control to move into different spinal shapes. While there are optimal positions that allow you to generate maximal force, other positions are not necessarily "unsafe." Normal movements require control, not avoidance. And the Deer movements help give you that control over your spine.

3. Monkey/Agility

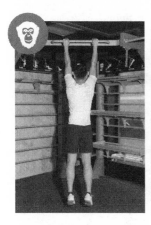 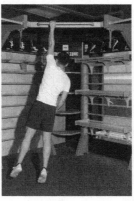 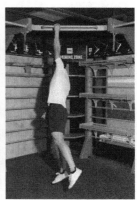

Imagine the spirit of a monkey: It should be full of energy, sneaky, and agile. Most of us had that spirit when we were young. We would climb onto things, sit on top of monkey bars, climb onto trees and rocks. Bring that curious spirit back and find your inner monkey!

The idea of the Monkey movement is to gain a pain-free range of motion in the thoracic spine (middle back) and improve shoulder function, thereby getting you or your athlete moving better overhead.

To do this movement, you will hold on to an overhead bar with both hands or one hand at a time, then sink your hips to lengthen the spine. When hanging by just one hand, you should turn the spine slightly so that the body must move through different planes. This involves the meridians and fascial lines listed in the following table.

MERIDIANS AND FASCIAL LINES INVOLVED IN THE MONKEY MOVEMENTS

Meridians	Fascial Lines
Lung and large intestine	Front
Pericardium and triple burner	Lateral
Heart, small intestine, gallbladder	Spiral

BENEFITS OF THE MONKEY MOVEMENT

Think of Roger Federer smashing that tennis ball during a serve, Michael Phelps outreaching competitors with his freestyle stroke, or Hall of Fame baseball pitcher Mariano Rivera closing out baseball games. Recognize any similarities between these sports? How are tennis, swimming, and baseball similar?

Many athletic movements, including the aforementioned ones, involve overhead components. Ironically, modern society is limiting many people's abilities to perform overhead movements effectively or efficiently. Put simply, people do not spend enough time where their arms are positioned over their head (quite the reverse, in fact—recall that insidious slouching posture). Over time, the lack of overhead movements creates structural or mechanical issues where joints and tissues are not functioning properly.

Weightlifting movements that include overhead components—the snatch and clean-and-jerk, for example—are seen as essential components of any modern strength and conditioning program because of the benefits associated with them: total body movement, coordination, strength, and power development.

But the overhead pressing pattern can get ugly quickly, and it's painful to watch. Athletes have a hard time establishing or maintaining proper positions. That's why athletes who do this kind of training often develop shoulder and lower back problems. Overhead pressing— or any overhead motion, in fact—requires multiple body parts to work in a synchronized way, including the middle back (thoracic spine), the shoulder blade (scapula), and the arm bone (humerus). The interaction between these three body parts determines how well an athlete is moving overhead.

Because athletes, like most humans today, are stuck in a hunched position (flexed middle back, protracted shoulder blades, and internally rotated shoulders), all three body parts may display limited range of motion when moving overhead. Remember the performance-deflating loop where the body develops new movement patterns from dysfunctions? In the case of raising both arms overhead, instead of extending the spine and opening the shoulders, the body compensates by overarching the lower back, which then leads to all sorts of problems.

As a way to reverse the performance-deflating loop, the Monkey movements involve *hanging* instead of pressing. One of the benefits of hanging is that the body is put in a good position where the arm bone is externally rotated, the shoulder blade is upwardly rotated and tilted toward the back, and the middle back is extended. With this combination of muscle and skeletal positions, the brain can relearn the proper way to put both arms overhead. The Monkey movements are also scalable, in that you can start by placing both feet on the ground and progress to taking both feet off the ground.

USING THE MONKEY MOVEMENTS TO BUILD CLIMBING STRENGTH

Most of us had no trouble climbing monkey bars, trees, or rocks during childhood. Yet climbing strength usually vanishes through adolescence. This is another classic example of "if you don't use it, you lose it!" After many years of non-movement, the body forgets how to climb efficiently.

Climbing movements are total body movements that rely on momentum and gravity. Hua Tuo highlighted climbing as one of the key characteristics of a monkey. While a human will not be able to climb as well as a monkey, climbing should be a natural ability that athletes have. Retrain the body to climb again and rediscover that strength that you naturally possess.

Upside-Down Monkey

The earliest descriptions of the Monkey series of movements in the Five Animal Frolics always included inversion (turning upside down). The idea is to get your head and torso positioned below your hips and legs, like a monkey hanging by its tail. In a gym, this is often done by using a hammock, as shown in the following image.

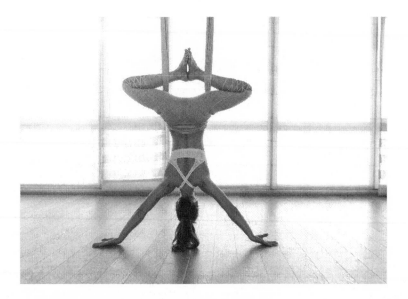

Hammock inversion with Monkey movement

The goal of inversion is to reverse the compression of gravity on the spine. Some of inversion's postulated benefits include increasing blood circulation, lymph drainage, and mobility and flexibility of the joints. We highly recommend adding inversion to your routine using whatever equipment you have available, such as draping your body over a hammock with the head hanging toward the ground or using inversion boots.

4. Crane/Elegance

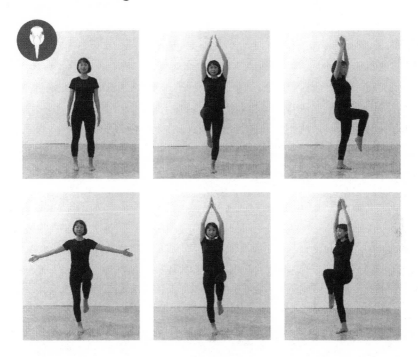

Cranes are long-legged birds, often found moving slowly through a marsh so they don't make waves in the water or holding a single position for long minutes as they wait for their prey to appear. The Crane movement helps build the balance and core strength needed to develop precise control over your own movements.

In the Crane series, you start in a standing position, then raise your arms over your head while simultaneously raising one leg. This involves the meridians and fascial lines shown in the following table.

MERIDIANS AND FASCIAL LINES INVOLVED IN CRANE MOVEMENTS

Meridians	Fascial Lines
Lung, heart, pericardium, large intestine, small intestine, spleen, stomach, and bladder	Arm
	Back
	Spiral

BENEFITS OF THE CRANE MOVEMENT:
BALANCE TRAINING

Balance is a component of all human movements. Proper balance requires optimal stability and postural control (through proprioceptive feedback—the body's awareness of where each of its parts is in space, as discussed on p. 53), which enhances performance and decreases the chances of injury. In sports, balance does not work in isolation, as it is combined with power, strength, speed, flexibility, mobility, and endurance. When performing the Crane, you can modify the intensity by changing variables such as speed and vision (eyes open to eyes closed).

5. Bear/Strength

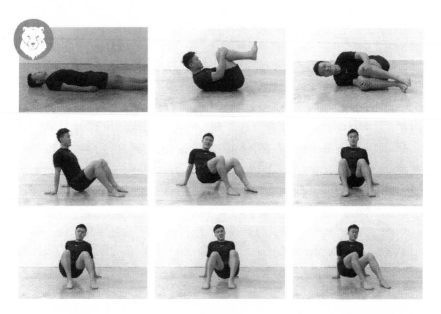

Bears are powerful creatures, so this series is designed to help build core muscle strength. The Bear movements are excellent for slouchers, because the movements require the exact opposite—a stretching of the front of the body rather than a compression of it.

To do the Bear, you start by lying down on the ground, then bringing your knees into your chest in a sort of hug and rocking from side to side. Then you will get into a seated position, with the arms straight behind you supporting the body (hands on the ground, palms facing away from the body) and feet flat on the ground. You then will raise the hips and rock slightly from side to side. This involves the meridians and fascial lines listed in the following table.

MERIDIANS AND FASCIAL LINES INVOLVED IN THE BEAR MOVEMENTS

Meridians	Fascial Lines
Lung, heart, large intestine, stomach, liver, and kidney	Arm lines

BENEFITS OF THE BEAR MOVEMENT: CHEST OPENER FOR BETTER POSTURE AND MOOD

The modern lifestyle is restless and mentally draining. If you are hunched over a computer, a bike, or your car's steering wheel all day, the length-tension relationship in your upper body will be affected and might result in a postural distortion known as upper-crossed syndrome: The head is migrated forward, and the shoulders are internally rotated. In severe cases, people might experience symptoms such as neck pain, headache, fatigue, and restricted movement.

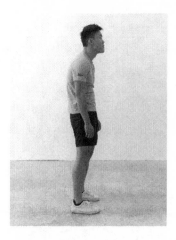

Example of slouched posture

From a TCM view, the slouching posture affects the lung meridian (shown in the following figure), the small intestine meridian, and the Ren meridian, also known as the Conception Vessel (not part of the classic twelve major channels). The lung meridian controls the breath and helps the heart in the circulation of blood. The small intestine meridian is linked to the heart, which helps modulate emotional health. The Ren meridian is linked to the Dan Tien, which is thought of as the ultimate powerhouse of the body. Even in Western culture, phrases such as "get it off my chest" associate the chest area with trapped emotions. Because of its role in opening the chest, the Bear movement should be an essential exercise for most modern people.

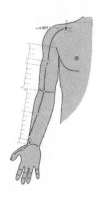

Lung Meridian

Improving Your Fascia through Movement

At the beginning of the chapter, we said that we would add another dimension to your training in the form of fascial training. To borrow the words of Dr. Robert Schleip and Divo Müller: "Of course, these fascia-oriented training suggestions should not replace muscular strength work, cardiovascular training and coordination exercises; instead, they should be thought of as a useful addition to a comprehensive training program."[8]

We do that by practicing an ancient movement routine created by Chinese surgeon Hua Tuo. The goal of Five Animal fitness is to grasp the awareness of a tiger, the gracefulness of a deer, the agility of a monkey, the elegance of a crane, and the strength of a bear. Countless variations of it have been included in dances, QiGong, and martial arts since its inception thousands of years ago.

The cool thing is that current research in exercise science supports ideas that were created two thousand years ago! Like many other historical figures who were credited with creating different movement routines, Hua Tuo had no intention of promoting himself as better than the others. Yet the Five Animal Movements are stunningly comprehensive. As you try out some of these movements at home, perhaps you will be like us, where we cannot help but appreciate the beauty and complexity of human movement.

---

8   Schleip R. and D. G. Müller. 2013. "Training Principles for Fascial Connective Tissues: Scientific Foundation and Suggested Practical Applications." *Journal of Bodywork and Movement Therapies* 17(1) (January): 103–15. doi: 10.1016/j.jbmt.2012.06.007. Epub 2012 Jul 21. PMID: 23294691.

INCORPORATING TCM RECOVERY TOOLS

At the beginning of this book, co-author Andy told the story of his early experience trying to bulk up in pursuit of his goal to play college-level soccer. Despite the early challenges he described, in 2014, Andy had the opportunity to try out for a professional soccer team. As you can imagine, this meant the world to him. "This was my dream growing up," Andy says, "and I was as close to the dream as ever."

Team practice sessions usually ran from 9:00 a.m. to 11:00 a.m. or 11:30 a.m., depending on whether there were individual drills to focus on after team practice. Apart from Wednesday afternoons, when a team gym session was mandatory, players were free to do whatever they wanted during the afternoons and evenings if there was not a game during the week. Some would take up coaching sessions, others would play video games, some would work out at the gym . . . and Andy? He would do some type of technique training in the afternoon, followed by gym sessions. He was focused on performance enhancement and desperate for a contract. He had to give his utmost effort. And here's Andy to tell the rest of the story:

It was a Monday session, which meant that practice was focused on conditioning for those who didn't play in the game during the weekend. It usually ended with eight to ten sprints of different variations. On that particular day, we did fifty-yard dashes. I had been doing quite well that day, beating my imaginary opponent, which was a teammate with similar speed. My plan was to really push to my limits for the last round.

The sprints were typically done with the starting players watching (Mondays were a recovery day for them if they had played in the match on the weekend). Those starting players would watch us, cheering us on or making subtle jabs, as one would in a team setting. So with the starters watching and myself on a trial, I was desperate to impress. I ran as fast as I could.

As I was approaching the finish line, I felt a tear in my right hamstring and had to stop running. I was devastated. Not so much because the injury hurt—although it did—but because my dream was effectively over.

This was my first valuable lesson on the importance of recovery. I had every reason to train hard every day, yet I overlooked the importance of rest and recovery. Because I never gave myself that time to relax, eventually my body gave up. And in this case, this cost me the chance to achieve my dream.

Andy's experience is an example of why we've said throughout this book that one of the main reasons to adopt TCM is to find ways to rebalance your life when something gets out of whack. In the previous three chapters, we talked about ways to help you maintain dynamic balance by incorporating TCM concepts into things you are already doing: your diet, breathing, and movement.

In this chapter, we want to talk about three TCM practices that you probably aren't doing already but that are known to help with recovery—which, as we discussed in the Introduction, is missing from most Western approaches to fitness and athletic performance. The physical and emotional toll imposed by hard workouts or competitions, and injuries large or small, can be balanced out by adopting techniques that help relieve pain, increase the flow of Qi and blood, and thus allow muscles and fascia to recover more quickly. The three specific recovery techniques we'll cover are the following:

1. **Cupping**—using cups or other devices to create a suction effect when placed on the skin. TCM uses it as a way to dispel stagnation, and in sports medicine, it is used as a soft tissue treatment to relieve pain, inflammation, and tension and improve circulation and relaxation.

2. **Gua Sha**—scraping a smooth-edged instrument across parts of the body. TCM uses it to release physical obstructions in the meridians and dispel toxins from the body. This method is used in sports medicine to detect fascial dysfunction; relieve pain, inflammation, and tension; and improve circulation and relaxation, similar to cupping.

3. **Acupuncture**—inserting thin needles into the body, usually along the meridians. It is used in TCM to stimulate the flow of Qi, treat pain, and provide mental stress relief.

Cupping: Restoring Balance to Muscles and Fascia

Ever since Olympian Michael Phelps appeared with dark purple circles around his shoulder region at the 2016 Olympic Games, cupping has become a hot topic among athletes.

Cupping is a treatment that, as the name implies, uses a cup to create suction on the skin over an area. You can think of it like a reverse massage—instead of pushing into the connective tissues (compression), the cup pulls (decompression). It is used by TCM practitioners and sports medicine professionals all over the world. Western-trained sports medicine professionals mainly use cupping as a technique to address strains or other minor injuries to the muscles, fascia, or other soft tissues. In China, though, the application of cupping is much broader; it includes treating soft tissue disorders but also removing toxins from the body and treating medical conditions such as coughing, asthma, the common cold, and even facial paralysis.

HISTORY OF CUPPING

Although cupping is an integral part of the TCM doctrine, the Chinese were not the first, nor the only, civilization to utilize this method, as it was also practiced in Egypt, ancient Greece, Macedonia, and the Middle East. This ancient method predates the written language, with the earliest records of usage found in the hieroglyphics of ancient Egypt.

The earliest record of cupping in China was included in *Wushi'er Bingfang* (Recipes for Fifty-Two Ailments), the first written medical text exclusively devoted to disease treatment. The text was compiled sometime between 1065 BC and 771 BC but was lost to history until it was rediscovered in 1973 during the excavation of an ancient tomb from the Han dynasty.

As cupping techniques evolved throughout the centuries, their therapeutic effects were recorded by TCM practitioners. Historically, cupping was used for suctioning harmful pus and treating pain, bites, pustules, headache, infections, and skin lesions. Some of the original instruments included animal horns, bones, bamboo, nuts, seashells, and gourds. As the technique continued to develop and evolve, cups were made from more durable materials, with size variations and different shapes.

Why Does Cupping Work?

We have identified three explanations, each from a different perspective, that explain the mechanisms of cupping.

1. **TCM:** Suction promotes the circulation of blood and Qi and removes waste products from the body.

2. **Mechanical:** Mechanical compression and suction to the local myofascial tissue (fascia surrounding the muscles) affects the tissue's viscoelasticity and stimulates other physiological responses.

3. **Neurophysiological:** Mechanical compression and suction to the local myofascial tissue influences tissue relaxation and pain reduction in the local and surrounding tissues through sensory input to the central nervous system.

OVERVIEW OF CUPPING TECHNIQUES

When you start investigating cupping techniques, the first thing you'll learn is that there are many different varieties based on factors such as the following:

- Cupping materials
- Suction methods
- Approach
- Dry vs. wet

Going into detail about the different types of cups and cupping practices is beyond the scope of this book, but we will discuss some of the more common variations, which are summarized in the following figure.

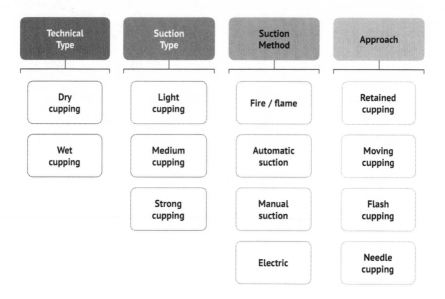

Common versions of cupping techniques

CUPPING MATERIALS

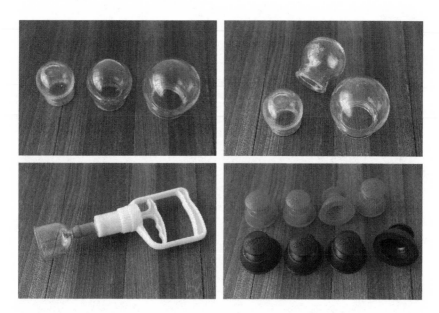

Throughout history, cupping was done using a region's local materials: animal horns, bamboo, ceramic, glass, metal, and plastic. Today, three types of material are commonly used:

- **Glass** is the most common material used in the TCM community because of hygienic reasons and its compatibility with fire (imagine adding fire to a plastic or silicone cup).

- **Plastic cups** are generally more portable and typically come with a pump suction device that can be applied with as much or as little pressure as preferred. The device can be manual or electric-powered.

- **Silicone cups** are convenient, don't require a pump, and offer the gentlest amount of suction. You just squeeze the cup and then apply it to the skin, similar to how you apply a phone mount to the windshield.

SUCTION METHODS

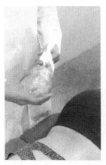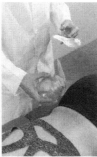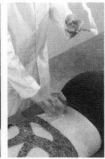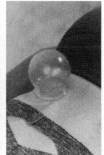

The essence of cupping is creating a suction effect. One way to do that is by allowing heated air to cool: Air expands as it is heated (which allows those giant balloons to rise into the atmosphere) and shrinks as it cools (which creates the suction effect). Another way to create a suction effect is through a pump that draws air out of the cup.

Using fire to heat up the air inside the cups is the most traditional method. In TCM, fire is viewed as an important aspect of the cupping treatment. Not only does fire create a better suction with glass cups, but fire cupping removes dampness from the body. (Remember, dampness is considered the cause or contributing factor to many illnesses.) Possible downsides to this method are risks associated with fire and not being able to control the level of suction.

Since plastic cups usually come with a suction pump that allows users to control the level of suction, this method is more popular with sports medicine professionals who are more focused on the level of myofascial decompression.

Silicone cups are easy to use and are good for targeting the superficial layers of connective tissues closer to the skin. Since the suction level is fixed and significantly less than that of a plastic or glass cup, it is not the ideal treatment for deep tissues.

CUPPING APPROACH

There are three basic cupping approaches, as summarized in the following chart.

THREE CUPPING APPROACHES

Approach	Description	Use/Outcomes
Retained Cupping	Cups are applied on a single site or along the myofascial lines or TCM meridians. TCM believes that this method helps dispel the cold and invigorates Qi and blood movement. Each cupping session typically lasts 8–10 minutes.	Retained cupping is commonly applied in treating muscle pain, soft tissue wounds, and sites with stagnation of Qi and blood—an example being slow-healing injuries.

Approach	Description	Use/Outcomes
Moving Cupping	The method is similar to re- tained cupping except the cup is dragged back and forth along myofascial lines or TCM merid- ians. Instead of remaining static, as with retained cupping, the effects of moving cupping seem to be more similar to Gua Sha (see p. 197).	Moving cupping is typically applied in treating sites with flat surfaces and that are large in size, such as the quadriceps, the abdomen, either side of the spine, and the shoulder region.
Flash Cupping	The basic technique is the same as for retained cupping except the cup is left on the site for just a brief moment, and the process is repeated a few times until the skin feels warm.	In addition to invigorating Qi and blood movement, flash cupping helps treat rheumatic diseases, untoned muscles, and skin numbness. It also alleviates post-stroke symptoms.

TYPE: DRY VS. WET CUPPING

When used alone, the term *cupping* generally refers to dry cupping: applying suction to the skin for a set time to achieve a therapeutic effect. As we've just discussed, traditional methods use fire to create a vacuum inside the glass cups, while modern methods use vacuum pumps to create suction.

Wet cupping includes a blood-letting process by cutting small inci- sions in the skin. We do not encourage such practice but wanted to include it in the book because it is a technique you may encounter. As this type of cupping involves blood, you must ensure that this is within your scope of practice and consult a licensed medical profes- sional before trying it.

HOW IS CUPPING USED?

Some practitioners may emphasize performing cupping on a precise site—an acupuncture point or along a meridian, for example. However, when we look at the historical records, different criteria have been used to determine where to place the cups—such as on sites of pain, discomfort, abnormal skin color, or abnormal skin temperature. In TCM there is a common saying that "*if the flow of Qi and blood is smooth, there is no pain; if the flow of Qi and blood is stagnated, there is pain.*" So cupping was intended to be a simple strategy to clear these "blockages" and alleviate pain and discomfort. There are no strict protocols on where and how many cups must be applied.

To best utilize cupping as a recovery technique, we advise that you get a movement assessment from a qualified movement specialist in addition to an assessment from a TCM practitioner to identify the areas that are most in need of improved circulation. Some common movement assessments include the Functional Movement Screen by Functional Movement Systems and the Three-Dimensional Movement Analysis & Performance System by the Gray Institute.

Cupping Tips

- Do not use cupping more than three to five times a week.

- Do not retain the cup for more than thirty minutes a session.

- Do not apply on the same site for consecutive days.

- There is no agreement on the right size of cup for different needs. You should use a cup that can cover most of the area you want to treat, without it falling off.

Gua Sha: Removing Obstructions and Blockages

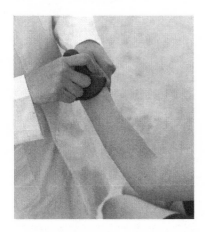
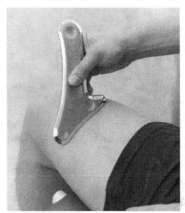

Gua Sha, also known as "scraping," "coining," and "spooning," is a technique that utilizes a smooth-edged instrument to repetitively scrape the skin and the underlying connective tissues. Like cupping, Gua Sha has been performed with different instruments: copper coins (hence the term *coining*), Chinese spoons (hence *spooning*), and even water buffalo horns, silver plate, and stones. Gua Sha was mainly a folk therapy for diseases and discomfort in China.

Kai Wen Tang, PhD, a registered TCM practitioner in Singapore, published a comprehensive book titled *Gua Sha: An Ancient Therapy for Contemporary Illnesses.* "In a nutshell," he writes, "Gua Sha is an ancient folk remedy in which the lubricated skin of the person seeking treatment is repeatedly 'press stroked' with a smooth-edged instrument in a methodical manner. . . . In so doing, stagnated energy is dissipated, blood flow improved, lymphatic circulation stimulated, inflammation reduced, and the body's physiological balance restored."[9]

In modern sports medicine, this technique is commonly referred to as instrument assisted soft tissue mobilization (IASTM). However,

---

9   Tang, K. W. 2020. *Gua Sha: An Ancient Therapy for Contemporary Illnesses.* Hackensack, NJ: World Scientific.

while IASTM is primarily used as a soft tissue treatment, Gua Sha is much broader in its application. Therefore, although the two methods share similarities in the form of scraping, Gua Sha is slightly different from IASTM.

HISTORY OF GUA SHA

It is uncertain whether Gua Sha actually originated in China, as roots can be traced to other Southeast Asian countries as well, where it has different names, including the following:

- Cambodia—*Kos Khyol*
- Indonesia—*Kerik*
- Thailand—*Hak*
- Vietnam—*Cạo Gió*

Written records of Gua Sha can be dated back to the Ming dynasty (1368–1644). However, it is believed that the treatment itself has been around for much longer.

To understand why and how the Chinese used this technique, we have to understand the meaning of Gua Sha: *Gua* translates to "scrape," while *Sha* translates to "sand" (Yes, sand!). But here it's not referring to those tiny granules you see at the beach. Instead, it refers to (1) the pattern of the reddish speckled rash on the skin after repetitive scraping, and (2) a philosophical concept that describes stagnant Qi and blood. Collectively, the goal of Gua Sha is to remove obstructions and toxins as strokes are applied through scraping.

HOW GUA SHA WORKS

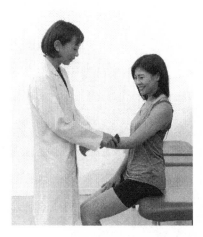

As with cupping, there are different explanations of how Gua Sha works, depending on which perspective you adopt:

1. **TCM:** to improve the flow of Qi and blood

2. **Mechanical:** to stimulate connective tissue remodeling through physically breaking down obstructions or adhesions in soft tissues

3. **Neurophysiological:** to stimulate the nervous system, creating changes in the neural drive to influence tissue tone and plasticity

Recall that stagnation in TCM can be an accumulation of Qi, blood, or waste body fluids (such as phlegm) due to a wide range of factors such as climate, season, dietary habits, dominance of one emotion, and extremes of movement (too much or too little). The act of scraping therefore physically breaks up the stagnation. Once the blocked passages and channels are cleared, the healthy Qi and blood can once again nourish the muscles, tissues, and substances in the targeted area. Think of our traffic network analogy in the chapter on the TCM meridians. Traditional Gua Sha is like an excavator; it is a fast way to destruct and dig up a messy site for the reconstruction of new infrastructures.

WHAT ABOUT THE RASHES?

If you look at pictures of people who have received a Gua Sha treatment, you will often see reddish speckled rashes or dots in the treated areas. These rashes or dots represent blood cells that have been pressed outside of capillaries (tiny blood vessels) as the practitioner repeatedly strokes the skin. The body begins the process of reabsorbing these blood cells immediately, and it is this process of reabsorption, along with a dramatic increase in local circulation, that results in the anti-inflammatory, immune-stimulating, and pain-relieving benefits of Gua Sha. Therefore, although these images may look scary and intimidating, they should not be confused with bruises (see the following table).

EFFECTS OF GUA SHA VS. BRUISING

Discoloration from Gua Sha	Bruise
Blood cells are pressed through the capillary wall without damage to the tissues.	Blunt force damages capillaries and causes bleeding into the tissue.

Acupuncture: Promoting Free Flow of Qi

Acupuncture is a treatment that involves the insertion of fine needles at specific points of the body, usually along the lines of meridians to promote free and unobstructed Qi. The method is used in treating various physical and mental conditions. Like cupping and Gua Sha, acupuncture is gaining popularity in sports medicine and is being used to treat various physical conditions.

In Chapter 1.3, on meridians, we mentioned that the meridian system is like a huge transport network. Inside this network are a number of stations called acupuncture points (acupoints). There are three predominant types of acupuncture points: meridian points, extra points, and ouch points (a-shi point). As with cupping and Gua Sha, there are different types of acupuncture, depending on which acupoints are targeted and the methodology used. The following table provides a summary of some common acupuncture types used for sports recovery.

COMMON ACUPUNCTURE TECHNIQUES FOR SPORTS RECOVERY

Type	Procedure	Common Symptoms and Condition Indications
Traditional Body Acupuncture	Insertion of fine needles through the skin at strategic sites on the body	• Musculoskeletal conditions • Pain conditions • Neurological conditions • Sleep conditions
Electro-Acupuncture	Traditional acupuncture connected to electrical stimulation equipment that induces different stimulation frequency, current intensity, pulse width, and pulse interval	Similar to traditional acupuncture, but studies have shown improvements in treating the following: • Post-stroke rehabilitation • Acute pain
Warm Needle Acupuncture	The combination of acupuncture with moxibustion (burning moxa, a cone or stick made of ground mugwort leaves) by placing a moxa stick on the handle of the acupuncture needle	In TCM terms: • Diseases that are Yin in nature • Yang Deficiency constitution
Sinew Acupuncture	Acupuncture without deep insertion of needles or the sore and numb sensation associated with traditional acupuncture; mostly performed on the outer layers of connective tissues closer to the skin	It is especially effective in treating acute pain and myofascial dysfunction.

HOW DOES ACUPUNCTURE WORK?

From a TCM perspective, the effectiveness of acupuncture is explained by its effect on the flow of Qi in the body.

From a modern scientific perspective, there is no universally accepted explanation. Numerous scientific studies have been undertaken to understand the mechanisms behind acupuncture. However, the mechanisms still remain unclear to modern scientists and researchers. Potential explanations include that acupuncture releases natural chemical messengers (neurotransmitters) that regulate pain and emotion and increase blood flow and metabolism.

DIY Acupressure Points

Applying pressure to and stimulating certain acupuncture points or meridians with your fingers or tools can produce a sore or numb sensation similar to the acupuncture experience. TCM practitioners believe that this sensation indicates the presence of *De-Qi* (which translates as "gained Qi") in the region or along the meridian. Let's put it this way: *De-Qi* can be used in alleviating meridian-related imbalances, because it is the ultimate goal of stimulating acupressure points through acupuncture.

Where's the Scientific Evidence?

From Michael Phelps's 2016 Olympic appearance to 2020, more than a dozen systematic reviews of original research—research that brings together all of the available evidence—were published on the topic of cupping. The results were inconsistent. Some studies showed an effect and others didn't. Why? Many researchers pointed to the lack of standardized research methods and the lack of quality design as the main contributing factors to inconsistent outcomes. A similar pattern can be seen if you review the scientific studies of Gua Sha and acupuncture:

- The scientific interest in these techniques—"scientific" in the modern interpretation of the word—is relatively new.

- There are few if any standards related to conducting scientific tests for these techniques.

- Applying the standard scientific method to the study of these techniques is difficult, because it is challenging to find placebos or other controls to compare them against.

- Because researchers do not yet know how to scientifically measure the outcomes, the treatments are often credited with only placebo effects or labeled as "pseudoscience."

Science is understanding the nature and behavior of natural things by unbiased observations and systematic experimentation. We agree that more scientific evidence—from a modern perspective—would help establish the effectiveness and mechanisms of cupping, Gua Sha, and acupuncture.

But we also want to acknowledge that "science" as we know it today has only existed for several hundred years, while TCM has been around for millennia. Each discipline developed a very different way to study and interpret the world. Yet neither can nor should claim to be superior to the other; it's quite possible that, in the future, TCM practitioners and trained scientists will find ways to collaborate on developing new methods to study and measure the effects of their recovery techniques. In the meantime, thousands of years of study and documentation by TCM practitioners should not be discounted.

One thing is for certain: The interest in these techniques is high and growing rapidly. What we have offered in this chapter are explanations of each technique and the evidence from history that supports their use.

Time for Recovery?

Ancient scholars and texts strongly advocated for the use of cupping and acupuncture. Ge Hong (283–343), who has been credited as the first user of cupping in China, popularized the saying that "more than half of the ills can be cured by acupuncture and cupping." Fast-forward to the modern day, and variations of cupping, Gua Sha, and acupuncture have spread all over the world. It's not hard to see why.

We talked in previous chapters about how fascia can become rigid and sticky, and used the term *fascial adhesion* to describe how rigid fascia has lost its smooth, sliding, and gliding capabilities. If that happens in your body, why not apply a tool that lifts (decompresses) the area that is stuck? Why not apply a technique that can physically identify those spots and alleviate them by applying smooth strokes? If you are struggling with stress, pain, and discomfort, why not try a natural and noninvasive approach that can calm you down and alleviate pain and discomfort?

The TCM philosophy stresses the importance of applying natural techniques for better well-being. As the research world continues to explore the underlying mechanisms of these methods, try out some of these techniques at home or visit your local licensed professional.

Don't Forget the Massage!

All of the techniques discussed in this chapter can be done in combination with massage to extend the therapeutic effects. You can also apply different self-massage products, such as a foam roller or massage gun, if you don't have access to a licensed massage therapist.

TO YOUR GOOD HEALTH

A s we've discussed throughout this book, the TCM definition of good health is to have balanced Qi—free from physical and emotional health issues. Good health is achieved not by striving for some ideal status but by establishing dynamic balance: the ability of your body to react to the onslaughts of daily life and rebalance when something shifts too far in any direction.

In Part 2, we talked about *reactive* steps you can take to address existing imbalances in your constitution and lifestyle. Here in Part 3 the focus was on *proactive* steps: changes you can make in your lifestyle to help maintain dynamic balance. These included the following:

1. Tailoring your diet to fit your constitution, the season, and the climate

2. Working on your breathing muscles and technique to improve the flow of Qi and counterbalance the negative impact of the stresses in your life

3. Adopting a warm-up or cooldown routine, such as the Five Animal Movements, that will help activate more muscles in your body and create more stability and mobility along the spine

4. Considering the use of one of the recovery techniques promoted by TCM (cupping, Gua Sha, and acupuncture)

To borrow the words of Wang Yongyan, who wrote in the *Journal of Traditional Chinese Medical Sciences* about exploring TCM through the lens of modern medical science, we believe these proactive steps "guard the root of life."

There is no magic bullet in traditional Chinese medicine that can instantaneously or dramatically enhance your performance. Rather, you will perform best when you follow the natural ways of living and when you follow the logical rules that guide the interactions of humans and nature.

PART 4

DEVELOPING YOUR OWN DYNAMIC BALANCE PLAN

STEPS TO CREATE YOUR OWN PLAN

Here we are at the final part of our journey. Our goal was to introduce the theoretical framework of TCM for you to apply to your lifestyle for better athletic performance. This part is where everything that we have discussed comes together. You will create your own performance-enhancement strategy using the seven steps that we have discussed in the book. Here is an overview of what you'll find in this section:

1. **Body constitution analysis (p. 74)**

   a. If you haven't already done so, complete the questionnaire to identify your constitution type. (You can refer to p. 69 if you filled out the original questionnaire, or use the one included in this part.)

2. **Diet analysis (p. 217)**

   a. Keep track of everything you eat and drink for three days (use the form on pp 218–220).

   b. Use the information in Appendix C to identify the dominant flavors and natures of the foods.

    c. Identify imbalances based on your body constitution, the season, your geographical location, and the flavors and natures of the foods.

    d. Use the information provided to identify changes you should consider to your diet.

3. **Emotional analysis (pp. 223–226)**

    a. Keep track of potential triggers of the fight-or-flight response.

    b. Think of ways to minimize or even eliminate unnecessary triggers.

4. **Fascia analysis (p. 229)**

    a. Use the form on pp. 229–230 or your preferred movement analysis to evaluate the status of your fascia.

    b. Ask a few guiding questions to examine why your fascia might not be able to maintain tensegrity.

    c. Use one or more techniques in steps 5–7 listed below (deep breathing, Five Animal Movements, TCM recovery tools).

    d. Incorporate these strategies into your plan so that you can regain and maintain the ease and fluidity that your fascia should have.

5. **Deep breathing exercise (p. 233)**

6. **The Five Animal Movements exercises (p. 237)**

    a. Tiger (p. 238)

    b. Deer (p. 241)

    c. Monkey (p. 244)

    d. Crane (p. 247)

    e. Bear (p. 250)

7. **Identifying which TCM recovery technique you may want to try (p. 253)**

YOUR BODY CONSTITUTION

Step 1: Complete the Constitution Questionnaire

If you completed this questionnaire in Part 2 (p. 69), you do not need to fill it out again. Skip to step 2.

QI DEFICIENCY

	Never	Seldom	Sometimes	Frequent	Always
Fatigued	1	2	3	4	5
Shortness of breath/panting (compared to people of your age)	1	2	3	4	5
Heart palpitations	1	2	3	4	5
Dizzy or lightheaded	1	2	3	4	5
Frequent colds and flu (especially when season changes)	1	2	3	4	5
Aloof and emotionally distant	1	2	3	4	5
Weak, breathy, or feeble voice	1	2	3	4	5
Excessive perspiration or night sweats	1	2	3	4	5
Total score divided by 8					

YANG DEFICIENCY

	Never	Seldom	Sometimes	Frequent	Always
Cold hands and feet/pale skin	1	2	3	4	5
Cold intolerance (sensitive to cold environments)	1	2	3	4	5
More layers of clothing than those around you	1	2	3	4	5
Chills in the abdomen, lower back, or knees	1	2	3	4	5
Prone to sickness/getting sick all the time (weak immune system)	1	2	3	4	5
Erectile dysfunction (male) or loss of sex drive (male or female)	1	2	3	4	5
Stomachache or diarrhea after eating cold/raw food and beverages	1	2	3	4	5
Repressed	1	2	3	4	5
Total score divided by 8					

YIN DEFICIENCY

	Never	Seldom	Sometimes	Frequent	Always
Warm or burning sensations in hands and feet (like to expose limbs or touch cool surfaces)	1	2	3	4	5
Feeling hot but no fever	1	2	3	4	5
Dry skin/cracked lips	1	2	3	4	5
Dark/burgundy-colored lips (natural state without makeup)	1	2	3	4	5
Constipation/dry hard stool	1	2	3	4	5
Redness/flushing of cheeks or face	1	2	3	4	5
Dry eyes	1	2	3	4	5
Dry mouth or constant thirst	1	2	3	4	5
Total score divided by 8					

PHLEGM-WETNESS

	Never	Seldom	Sometimes	Frequent	Always
Chest tightness/ abdominal bloating	1	2	3	4	5
Heaviness in limbs and body/lethargic	1	2	3	4	5
Delayed or slow bowel movements	1	2	3	4	5
Oily forehead	1	2	3	4	5
Puffy eyes	1	2	3	4	5
Mouth feels sticky	1	2	3	4	5
Excessive mucus in throat	1	2	3	4	5
Thick tongue coating	1	2	3	4	5
Total score divided by 8					

WETNESS-HEAT

	Never	Seldom	Sometimes	Frequent	Always
Oily face/nose	1	2	3	4	5
Prone to acne	1	2	3	4	5
Bitter/bad taste in mouth	1	2	3	4	5
Sticky stool/tenesmus (sensation of needing to pass stool)	1	2	3	4	5
Hot or burning urine/dark urine (dark like amber)	1	2	3	4	5
Yellow discharge (female only)	1	2	3	4	5
Sweaty testicles (male only)	1	2	3	4	5
Total score divided by 6					

BLOOD STASIS

	Never	Seldom	Sometimes	Frequent	Always
Petechiae/ecchymosis (unexplained bruising without bumping into things)	1	2	3	4	5
Rashes on face	1	2	3	4	5
Body aches	1	2	3	4	5
Dull skin tone	1	2	3	4	5
Dark circles under the eyes	1	2	3	4	5
Poor memory/forgetfulness	1	2	3	4	5
Dark red or purple lips (natural state without makeup)	1	2	3	4	5
Total score divided by 7					

QI STAGNATION

	Never	Seldom	Sometimes	Frequent	Always
Depressed or unmotivated	1	2	3	4	5
Anxiety/frustration	1	2	3	4	5
Emotional and sensitive	1	2	3	4	5
Easily frightened/fearful	1	2	3	4	5
Mastalgia (breast pain for women)/ discomfort around the sides of rib cage (both men and women)	1	2	3	4	5
Sighing	1	2	3	4	5
Sensation of lump in the throat	1	2	3	4	5
Total score divided by 7					

BALANCED HEALTH

	Never	Seldom	Sometimes	Frequent	Always
Easily fatigued	5	4	3	2	1
Weak/breathy voice	5	4	3	2	1
Constantly feeling down or gloomy	5	4	3	2	1
Cold aversion (including to AC or fans in summer)	5	4	3	2	1
Sensitive to natural changes in the environment (climate, weather)	5	4	3	2	1
Insomnia	5	4	3	2	1
Forgetful	5	4	3	2	1
Total score divided by 7					

Step 2: Summarize the Results from the Questionnaire

Write down the average score for each section of the questionnaire.

Constitution	Average Score
Qi Deficiency	
Yang Deficiency	
Yin Deficiency	
Phlegm-Wetness	
Wetness-Heat	
Blood Stasis	
Qi Stagnation	
Balanced Health	

Step 3. Identify Your Dominant Constitution Type(s) and Its Characteristics

Which type(s) received your biggest score in the summary table?

_____

_____

_____

_____

(If you have two or more scores that are close, list each type.)

Refer to the table on constitution types in Chapter 2.1 (p. 75) and jot down notes that relate to your constitution type. We've left room for multiple constitutions in case you have two or three that score high:

Constitution Type	Characteristics (from the Body Constitution Questionnaire in Chapter 2.1)

Step 4. What Do You Think This Means for You?

What insights have you gained from your body constitution analysis?

_____

_____

_____

_____

_____

_____

DIET ANALYSIS

In this section, you will document what you eat and drink for three days, then analyze the flavors and natures of those foods. You can see how we completed a diet analysis by referring to the evaluation of our case study of Ben's diet in Appendix E and on pp. 102–105 in Chapter 2.3.

Step 1: Document What You Eat and Drink

Use the following form to write down everything you eat and drink for three days. When you're done, use Appendix C to analyze the flavor and nature of each item.

DAY 1

Time	Name and portion of food/drink (roughly)	Flavor(s)	Nature

DAY 2

Time	Name and portion of food/drink (roughly)	Flavor(s)	Nature

DAY 3

Time	Name and portion of food/drink (roughly)	Flavor(s)	Nature

Step 2. Summarize the Results

Add up the number of each flavor and nature for each day of your diet journal. Enter the numbers below, then total each column.

| | FLAVOR | | | | | NATURE | | | | |
| | | | | | | Yin ⟵ | | | ⟶ | Yang |
	Sour	Sweet	Bitter	Spicy	Salty	Cold	Cool	Neutral	Warm	Hot
Day 1										
Day 2										
Day 3										
TOTAL										

Step 3. Document Your Location, the Season, and the Climate

Where are you located?	
What is the current season?	
What is the climate?	

Step 4. Determine Your Dietary Direction

Think about your dominant body constitution type(s), the season, and the climate. The following table summarizes the key dietary guidance for each constitution type (you can find details about which foods to eat and which to avoid in Appendix D).

SUMMARY OF DIETARY STRATEGIES ACCORDING TO BODY CONSTITUTION

Constitution	Strategy
Qi Deficiency	Eat foods that nourish the spleen and the gut.
Yang Deficiency	Eat foods that are neutral, warm, and nourishing.
Yin Deficiency	Eat foods that are neutral, cool, and nourishing to clear deficient heat. Avoid stimulating foods and drinks. Avoid dehydrating food.
Phlegm-Wetness	Eat foods to nourish the spleen and to clear phlegm and dampness. Avoid raw, cold, oily, and heavily processed foods.
Wetness-Heat	Eat nourishing and cool foods or food that can increase urination to expel excessive heat and dampness from the body.
Qi Stagnation	Eat foods that stimulate Qi.
Blood Stasis	Eat foods that stimulate blood.
Balanced Health	No changes needed. Eat a variety of foods. Stay in balance!

Given all this information, in what ways is your diet out of balance? What types of food and beverages should you consume or avoid to make it more balanced?

_____

_____

_____

ANALYSIS OF YOUR EMOTIONAL BALANCE AND STRESS LEVELS

A s you may recall from Chapter 2.4, some emotions are considered positive and others negative. But neither type is all good or all bad—the question is whether you allow any of them to dominate your life. Dynamic balance doesn't mean you won't have an excess of emotions sometimes. It means you learn to recognize when certain emotions are too dominant, and develop strategies for coming back into balance.

Which Emotions Lead to Imbalance for You?

Review the following table (repeated from Chapter 2.4, which summarizes the emotions from a TCM point of view).

Which of these emotions give you the most trouble in terms of their excess?

Emotion	Yin-Yang	Governed by	Movement of Qi	Symptoms of Excess
Anger	Yang	Liver	Rises	• Headaches • Dizziness • Forgetfulness • Tensed muscles
Joy	Yang	Heart	Slows	• Insomnia • Disorientation
Worry/ Pensiveness	Yin	Spleen	Stagnates	• Bloating • Loss of appetite • Poor concentration • Menstrual cycle disruption
Anxiety	Yin	Lungs	Stagnates	• Gasping • Tight sensation in chest • Constipation • Fatigue
Melancholy/ Grief/ Sadness	Yin	Lungs	Depletes	• Shortness of breath • Congested nose • Muscle spasms • Rib cage pain
Fear	Yin	Kidney	Descends	• Urinary incontinence • Muscle atrophy • Hair loss • Pain in bones and joints • Erectile dysfunction
Fright	Yang	Kidney	Scatters	• Indecisiveness • Palpitations • Feeling stunned • Insane behavior

_____

_____

_____

_____

_____

_____

Fight-or-Flight Triggers

One of the most common problems in today's world is how much *unnecessary* stress and anxiety we all experience every day. The constant triggering of our fight-or-flight response causes a cascade of problems that lead to imbalances, as we discussed in Chapter 2.4.

If you filled out this table in Chapter 2.4, just copy the numbers from there.

POSSIBLE FIGHT-OR-FLIGHT TRIGGERS

Events	Time Spent (hours/minutes)
Traffic jam	
Crowded environment	
Work-related stress	
School-related stress	
Home-related stress	
Cell phone use	
Video streaming/TV watching	
Total	

DIGGING DEEPER INTO CELL PHONE USE

While smartphones have had a revolutionary impact on society, Steve Jobs did not create the iPhone with the intention of making it an addiction. Nowadays, people are spending way too much time on their smartphones looking for love (dating apps), winning social acceptance (social media), achieving status and honor (video games), and being entertained (video platforms). Your phone records everything that you do and how much time you spend doing it. Open the screen time tab that gives you the daily average time that you have spent on your phone. Now write down the total amounts for your five most-used apps from last week.

DAILY AVERAGE SCREEN TIME FOR THE WEEK OF:

Top 5 most-used apps and time spent on each:	
1.	
2.	
3.	
4.	
5.	

Now, explain to yourself why you needed to spend so much time on those apps.

_____

_____

_____

_____

_____

Most people have a hard time justifying why they need to spend an hour on Instagram every day, given that their job isn't to manage social media. While there are instances when the phone is a helpful tool, too much smartphone usage will unsettle our brain. Jim Kwik, an expert in brain health, even goes so far as to suggest ditching the smartphone for a smarter brain. Should we? You should know our views by now, hopefully. No—because balance is key.

Just be mindful of how you might be tricking yourself into fight-or-flight mode.

Embrace the Boredom

Georgetown University professor Cal Newport has a brilliant strategy that could help the modern-day athlete who is struggling with their smartphone use, and he shared the strategy in the *Wall Street Journal* bestselling book *Deep Work*—embrace boredom. You see, the deeper problem behind spending too much time on TikTok or Instagram is that our brains are constantly looking for stimulation (Yang). But as Newport pointed out, our brains cannot be working hard all the time. The brain needs time to be bored (Yin) to recover, and boredom is crucial because that's when creative ideas come to mind.

So the next time you are waiting for your meal to arrive, commuting to practice, or taking a break at work, know that a little boredom is good for you, and embrace the opportunity to be that odd person not scrolling and swiping on their screen.

Your Plan

Think about how much time you spend in the Yang state: excited, anxious, stressed. Is there enough Yin in your life? Are you giving your brain enough time to rest and recover?

One tip is to try and embrace boredom while you are waiting for your meal this week. Work on your breathing instead! Write down your own ideas for creating more calmness in your life:

_____

_____

_____

_____

_____

HOW HEALTHY IS YOUR FASCIA?

The TCM concept of balanced health is predicated on the idea of smooth and unobstructed Qi-blood circulation throughout the body. A key area that must be considered is the fascial system. We have identified three factors that influence the health of the fascial system: posture, diet, and emotions.

To see if your posture and movement (or lack thereof) are making your fascia too rigid, we suggest you complete the following worksheet where you can reflect on whether your daily lifestyle is reinforcing rigid fascia.

Fascial Health Worksheet

1. Does your daytime activity (work/studying) require you to sit or stand still for prolonged periods of time? If yes, estimate the time you spend in any single position during the day.

   _____

   _____

2. What types of repetitive movements are required for your sport or activity?

_____

_____

_____

3. Rate the fluidity of your movements on a scale of 1 (poor) to 10 (excellent). Are you smooth and elegant or rigid and tight?

Rigid, tight							Smooth, elegant		
1	2	3	4	5	6	7	8	9	10

4. How much time every day are you exposing yourself to potential fight-or-flight situations? (See the Fight-or-Flight Triggers worksheet in Chapter 4.3, p. 115.)

_____

_____

_____

5. How much water (coffee, tea, and juice do not count) are you drinking per day? Do you think it's enough, too little, or too much?

_____

_____

_____

Action Tips

Your body is not made to be static and stationary; it is made to move. If you find yourself being static the entire day sitting in front of a computer, *set a timer to move every half hour to forty-five minutes.* You don't have to do a full workout, but if you are forced to sit most of the day, go to the kitchen, get some water (not tea, not coffee, not juice), and stretch the front lines of the body. If you stand a lot, use the timer to remind yourself to bend and stretch, and even sit for a few minutes if possible.

Talk with your strength and conditioning coach for a needs analysis for the sport you play—it examines the predominant movements that your sport requires. Determine which muscles are prone to overuse injuries. Reverse the performance-deflating loop by stretching or massaging those muscles after training.

If you are a rigid mover, know that this could happen because you are in a fight-or-flight mode all day, and you might not be drinking enough water. Your fascia is like a sponge that is drained of water. Drink water to hydrate your tissues. Utilize that water break to enjoy some light movement, embrace boredom for a few minutes, and work on your breathing!

Your Fascia Action Plan

What ideas do you have to incorporate more movement and flexibility into your day?

_____

_____

_____

_____

STRENGTHEN YOUR BREATHING

Strengthen your breathing by being mindful of how you breathe. Incorporate the following breathing practice to help calm your mental state. This can be done while you are in an elevator, waiting to cross the road, or even before an important game!

1. Be mindful of the five body checkpoints to make sure the body is in proper alignment, as shown in the following figure (head, shoulders, hips, knees, and feet in alignment).

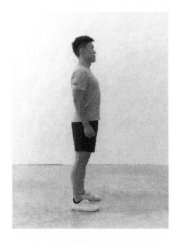

2. Place one hand on the chest and the other on the abdomen. If
   you think this makes you look odd in public, then just use two
   imaginary hands instead.

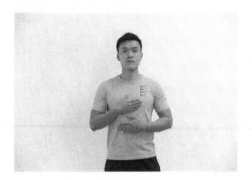

3. Take deep nasal breaths (in through the nose) and exhale out
   of the mouth.

4. The hand on the abdomen should move first, and the most.
   The hand on the chest should move minimally.

5. Repeat this process a few times for however much time
   is allowed.

Upgrade Your Core Workout to Incorporate Deep Breathing

Dr. Stuart McGill, a world-renowned expert on spinal health whom we introduced in Chapter 3.2, found that three specific core exercises—the curl-up, side
plank, and bird-dog (known as "The Big 3")—target all areas of the spine without placing excessive stress on the parts of the back that are prone to injury.
You can find detailed descriptions of these exercises on the internet. Here's
how you can upgrade them to include breathing work:

1. **Curl-up:** You exhale when curling up and inhale when lowering the body back to the ground. *Upgrade:* Spend some time in the transition period (the time when your body is in the air) to work on full belly breaths.

2. **Side plank:** Typically done with shallow breaths or even no breaths (during the last few seconds). *Upgrade:* Take deep belly breaths throughout those thirty seconds (or however long you set the timer for).

3. **Opposite leg and arm raise (bird-dog):** In this exercise, you raise one arm and the opposite leg at the same time until they are parallel to the ground, then repeat the movement with the opposite pair. *Upgrade:* Once you get to that parallel point, hold that position, take a deep breath, inhale, and then return to the start on the exhale.

Breathing Action Plan

Use the space below to write down your ideas for how you can add the preceding breathing exercise into your everyday routine, and how you can be more mindful of deep breathing during your workouts.

FIVE ANIMAL MOVEMENTS EXERCISES

If you want to try incorporating the Five Animal Movements into your fitness routine, here are some tips to get you started:

- The Five Animal Movements practice can be part of a warm-up, a cooldown, or a standalone workout.

- The pace of movement should be slow (unless you want to use it as an aggressive warm-up, then you will go fast), as we are focusing on elongating the soft tissues of the body.

- If you do all five movements, you don't need to follow the specific order that we use here. Do what is right for your body.

- You can also choose to focus on a subset of the series. For example, work on the Crane if you struggle with balance or the Bear if you struggle with a slouching posture.

- Approach the five movements with an explorer mentality, and have fun—after all, they were called "frolics" not "robotic drills"!

- As you go through the steps, explore a comfortable range of movement. If you feel any discomfort, ease back to a comfortable position or stop the movement.

1. Tiger Instructions

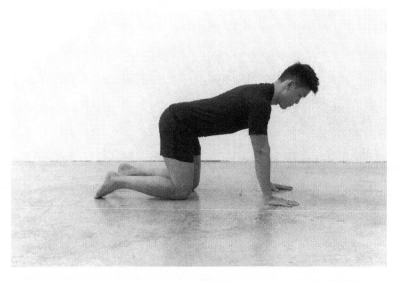

1. Begin in a quadrupedal position: hands and knees on the ground, with the feet shoulder-width apart. Lift the knees off the ground while maintaining a slight knee bend.

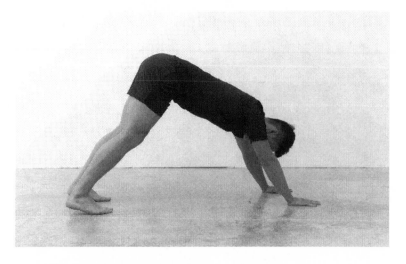

2. Pull your hips toward the sky.

3. Push your arms into the ground.

4. Take one full belly breath.

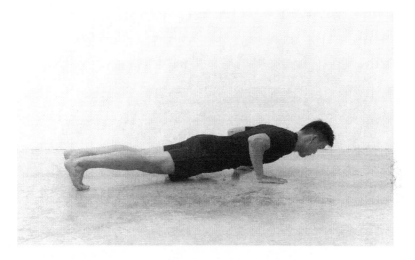

5. Lower your head and chest without touching the ground.

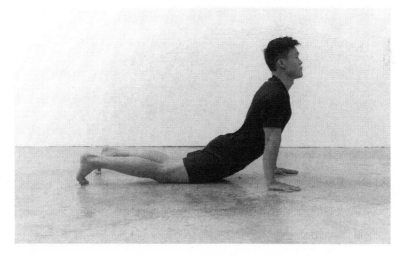

6. Raise the upper body up toward the ceiling.

7. Take one full belly breath.

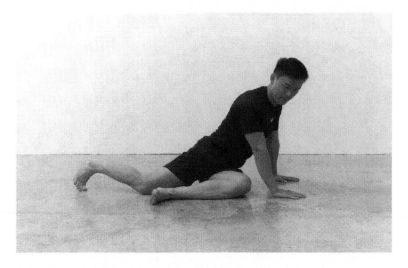

8. Cross the left knee over to the right side while maintaining a 90-degree knee bend.

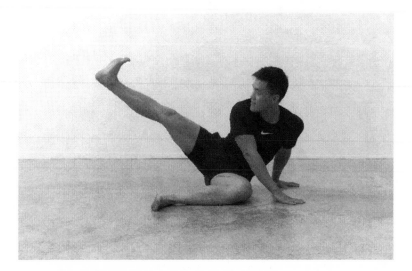

9. Raise the left leg.

10. Take one full belly breath.

11. Lower the left leg and repeat on the other side.

12. Return to the standard Tiger position.

13. Repeat steps 1 to 12 seven times.

Common Faults with the Tiger

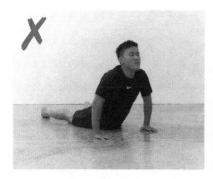 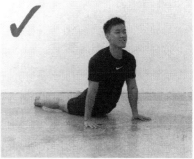

Raised shoulders

Elbows flaring out

Keep the shoulders down

Elbow pits facing forward

2. Deer Instructions

1. Start in a quadrupedal position.

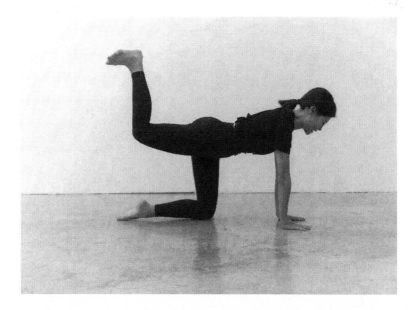

2. Lift your right leg off the ground.

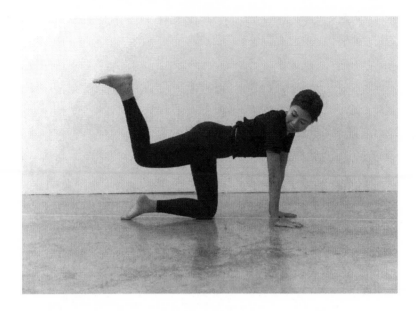

3. Rotate your right thigh internally so that the right heel is outside the body.

4. Tilt your spine laterally to the right.

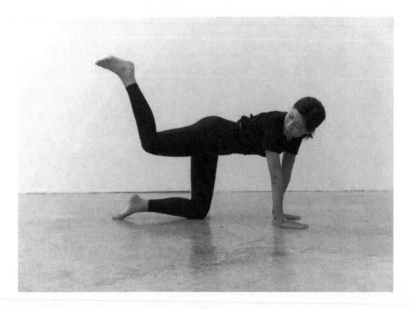

5. Turn your head to the right, mimicking a deer checking its surroundings.

6. Take one full belly breath.

7. Repeat steps 1 to 6 on the left side.

8. Perform these seven times on each side.

Common Faults with the Deer

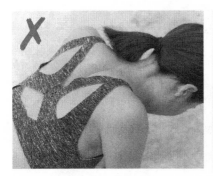

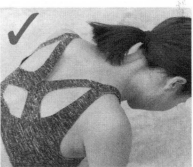

Shoulder blades
passively hanging

Shoulder blades actively
pushing into the ground

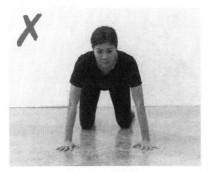

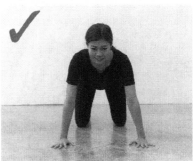

Elbow pits facing inward

Elbow pits facing forward

3. Monkey Instructions

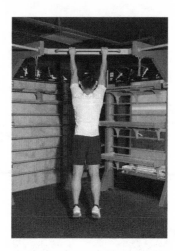

1. Hold on to a bar with an overhand closed grip (feet off the floor).

2. Straighten the arms.

3. Relax and let the shoulders come up by the ears.

4. Hang for one full belly breath.

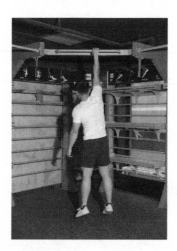

5. Hang using the right arm only.

6. Take one full belly breath.

7. Hang using the left arm only.

8. Take one full belly breath.

9. Regression: If hanging is too challenging, have the legs maintain contact with the floor so they can function as a support.

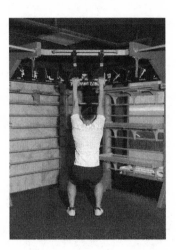

Common Faults with the Monkey

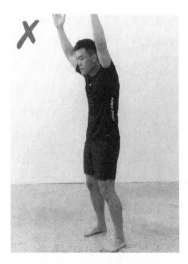

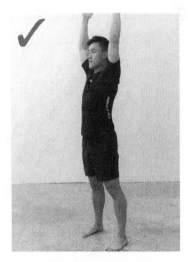

Head migrated forward	Head in neutral position
Rounded shoulders	Shoulders in neutral position

4. Crane Instructions

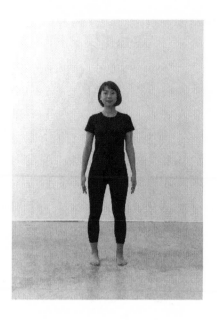

1. Start in a standing position. Knees and toes should be pointing in the same direction (forward).

2. Raise both arms overhead.

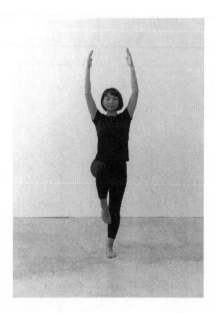

3. Lift the right leg off the ground.

4. Take one full belly breath.

5. Lower the arms to shoulder height, with palms facing forward.

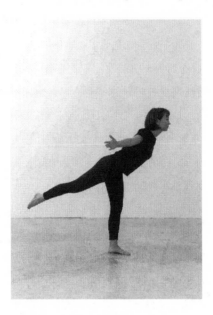

6. Kick the right leg back.

7. Take one full belly breath.

8. Repeat steps 2 to 7 with the left leg.

9. Perform these seven times on each side.

Common Faults with the Crane

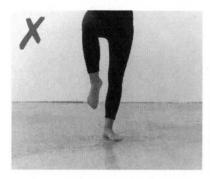

Feet turned out

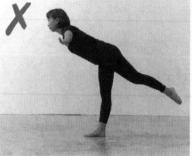

Feet turned in

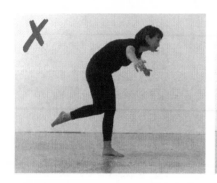

Bending from lower back

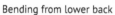

Locked knee

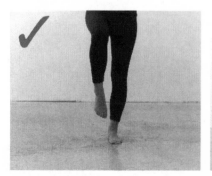

Knees and toes aligned

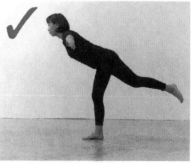

Squared hips and knees slightly bent

5. Bear Instructions

1. Start by lying on the floor.

2. Take one full belly breath.

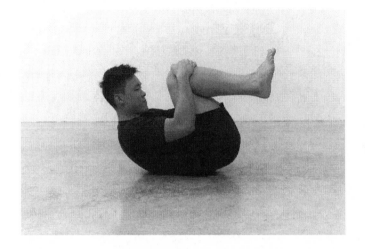

3. Hug both knees with the arms.

4. Take one full belly breath.

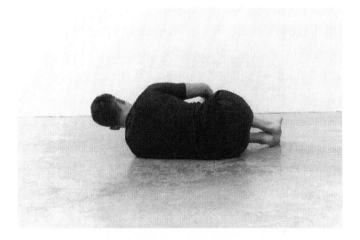

5. Rock the body from one side to the other until the side of the body touches the ground.

6. Return to the starting lying position.

7. Sit up so that the upper body is tilted at an angle.

8. Place the arms behind the body, fingers pointing away from the body.

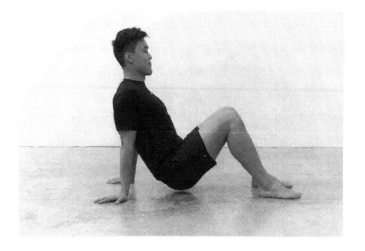

9. Lift the hips off the ground.

10. Take one full belly breath.

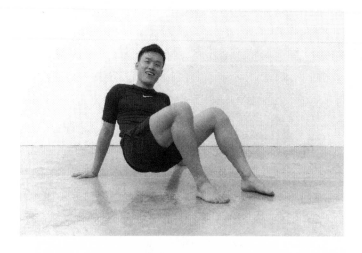

11. Rock from side to side for seven repetitions.

Common Faults with the Bear

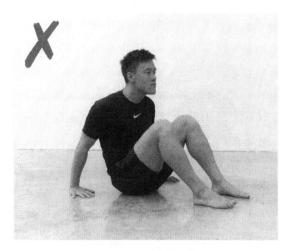

Fingers pointing toward the body

Head migrated forward

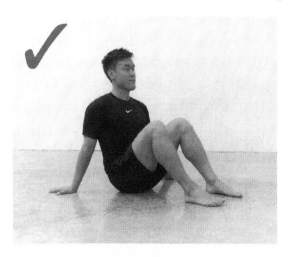

Shoulders externally rotated

Head in neutral position

RECOVERY TECHNIQUES

The following table summarizes the recovery techniques discussed in Chapter 3.4.

Technique	What It Does	Useful for
Cupping	The cups produce a suction effect to lift and decompress layers of connective tissues.	Relieving areas that are prone to overuse, as determined by a needs analysis
Gua Sha	A smooth-edged instrument removes physical obstructions through rhythmic strokes.	Detecting unhealthy fascia and alleviating "knots" as a result of overuse
Acupuncture*	Thin needles are inserted into different acupuncture points to stimulate circulation.	Improving metabolism, managing stress, and alleviating pain
Massage	Pressure is applied to different parts of the body to relieve tension or discomfort.	Relaxing the tissues, increasing circulation, and calming the mind

*Make sure you visit a licensed professional.

Based on the analysis of your own body constitution, lifestyle, and current imbalances, which recovery technique would you want to try first? Why? What results would you hope to see?

_____

_____

_____

_____

_____

APPENDICES

APPENDIX A

BIBLIOGRAPHY

Part 1: Essential Chinese Medicine Concepts

1.1 The Vital Substances of Life (Qi and Blood)

1. Beinfield, H. and E. Korngold. 1991. *Between Heaven and Earth: A Guide to Chinese Medicine.* New York: Random House Publishing Group.

2. Fu, J. and M. Yang. 2019. *The Yellow Emperor's Classic of Medicine: Essential Questions.* Singapore: World Scientific Publishing.

3. Maciocia, G. 2005. *The Foundations of Chinese Medicine.* Edinburgh: Elsevier Churchill Livingstone.

4. Tang, K. W. 2020. *Gua Sha: An Ancient Therapy for Contemporary Illnesses.* Hackensack, NJ: World Scientific.

5. Taylor, S. 2014. "Chinese Medicine Demystified Part 2—What Is Qi?" Retrieved December 23, 2020, from https://acupuncturesanantonio.com/chinese-medicine-demystified-part-2-qi.

1.2 The Language of Balance and Harmony (Yin-Yang and Five Phases)

1. Fu, J. and M. Yang. 2019. *The Yellow Emperor's Classic of Medicine: Essential Questions.* Singapore: World Scientific Publishing.

2. Maciocia, G. 2005. *The Foundations of Chinese Medicine.* Edinburgh: Elsevier Churchill Livingstone.

1.3 The Body Is Not a Machine (Zang-Fu and Meridians)

1. Beinfield, H. and E. Korngold. 1991. *Between Heaven and Earth: A Guide to Chinese Medicine.* New York: Random House Publishing Group.

2. Fu, J. and M. Yang. 2019. *The Yellow Emperor's Classic of Medicine: Essential Questions.* Singapore: World Scientific Publishing.

3. Maciocia, G. 2005. *The Foundations of Chinese Medicine.* Edinburgh: Elsevier Churchill Livingstone.

1.4 The Search for Smooth and Eloquent Movements (Muscles and Fascia)

1. Bai, Y., J. Wang, J. Wu, J. Dai, O. Sha, D. T. Yew, Q. Liang, et al. 2011. "Review of Evidence Suggesting That the Fascia Network Could Be the Anatomical Basis for Acupoints and Meridians in the Human Body." *Evidence-Based Complementary and Alternative Medicine* 1–6. doi:10.1155/2011/260510.

2. Bodybuildingcom. 2020. "What Is the Best 5-Day Workout Split?" October 23, 2020. Retrieved December 26, 2020, from https://www.bodybuilding.com/content/what-is-the-best-5-day-workout-split.html.

3. Bordoni, B. and F. Marelli. 2017. "Emotions in Motion: Myofascial Interoception." *Complementary Medicine Research* 24(2): 110–113. doi:10.1159/000464149.

4. Gómez-Jáuregui, V. 2010. *Tensegrity Structures and their Application to Architecture.* Servicio de Publicaciones Universidad de Cantabria. 19. ISBN 978-8481025750.

5. Langevin, H. M. 2006. "Connective Tissue: A Body-Wide Signaling Network?" *Medical Hypotheses* 66(6): 1074–1077. doi:10.1016/j.mehy.2005.12.032.

6. McCall, P. 2013. "Cutting Edge: Training the Fascial Network (Part 1)." April 2013. Retrieved December 30, 2020, from https://www.acefitness.org/certifiednewsarticle/3161/cutting-edge-training-the-fascial-network-part-1.

7. Myers, T. 2009. *Anatomy Trains* (2nd ed.). London: Elsevier.

8. Norlyk Smith, E. 2014. "Creating Change: Tom Myers on Yoga, Fascia

and Mind-Body Transformation." February 5, 2014. Retrieved December 26, 2020, from https://www.huffpost.com/entry/mind-body-_b_4387093.

9. Schleip R. and D. G. Müller. 2013. "Training Principles for Fascial Connective Tissues: Scientific Foundation and Suggested Practical Applications." *Journal of Bodywork and Movement Therapies* 17(1) (January): 103–15. doi: 10.1016/j.jbmt.2012.06.007. Epub 2012 Jul 21. PMID: 23294691.

10. Schleip, R. and J. Wilke. 2021. *Fascia in Sport and Movement.* Pencaitland: Handspring Publishing.

11. Schultz, R. L. and Feitis, R. 1996. *The Endless Web: Fascial Anatomy and Physical Reality.* Berkeley, CA: North Atlantic Books.

12. Van Der Wal, J. 2009. "The Architecture of the Connective Tissue in the Musculoskeletal System—An Often Overlooked Functional Parameter as to Proprioception in the Locomotor Apparatus." *International Journal of Therapeutic Massage & Bodywork: Research, Education, & Practice* 2(4). doi:10.3822/ijtmb.v2i4.62.

Part 1 Debrief: Piecing Together the East and the West

1. Wang, J. 2012. "Traditional Chinese Medicine and The Positive Correlation with Homeostatic Evolution of Human Beings: Based on Medical Perspective." *Chinese Journal of Integrative Medicine* 18(8), 629–634. doi:10.1007/s11655-012-1170-3.

Part 2: Seeking Sources of Imbalance and Fatigue

2.1 What Is Your Body Constitution Type?

1. Sun, Y., Y. Zhao, S. A. Xue, and J. Chen. 2018. "The Theory Development of Traditional Chinese Medicine Constitution: A Review." *Journal of Traditional Chinese Medical Sciences* 5(1), 16–28. https://doi.org/10.1016/j.jtcms.2018.02.007.

2. Wang, Q. 1995. *Traditional Chinese Medicine Constitutionology [Chinese]*. Beijing: China Medical Science Press.

3. Wang, Q., Y. B. Zhu, H. S. Xue, and S. Li. 2006. "Primary Compiling of Constitution in Chinese Medicine Questionnaire." *Chinese Journal of Clinical Rehabilitation* 10(3), 12–14.

4. Wong, W., C. L. Lam, V. T. Wong, Z. M. Yang, E. T. Ziea, and A. K. Kwan. 2013. "Validation of the Constitution in Chinese Medicine Questionnaire: Does the Traditional Chinese Medicine Concept of Body Constitution Exist?" *Evidence-Based Complementary and Alternative Medicine* 1–14. doi:10.1155/2013/481491.

2.3 An Imbalance in Diet Depends on Your Situation

1. Brietzke, C., P. E. Franco-Alvarenga, H. J. Coelho-Júnior, R. Silveira, R. Y. Asano, and F. O. Pires. 2018. "Effects of Carbohydrate Mouth Rinse on Cycling Time Trial Performance: A Systematic Review and Meta-Analysis." *Sports Medicine* 49(1), 57–66. doi:10.1007/s40279-018-1029-7.

2. Carter, J. M., A. E. Jeukendrup, and D. A. Jones. 2004. "The Effect of Carbohydrate Mouth Rinse on 1-h Cycle Time Trial Performance." *Medicine and Science in Sports and Exercise*, 36(12), 2107–2111. https://doi.org/10.1249/01.mss.0000147585.65709.6f.

3. Dharmananda, S. 2010. "Taste and Action of Chinese Herbs—Traditional and Modern Viewpoints." October 2010. Retrieved from http://www.itmonline.org/articles/taste_action/taste_action_herbs.htm.

4. Haff, G. and N. T. Triplett. 2016. *Essentials of Strength Training and Conditioning*. Champaign, IL: Human Kinetics.

5. Hantzidiamantis, P. J. and S. L. Lappin. 2020. *Physiology, Glucose*. Updated August 13, 2019. In: StatPearls [Internet]. Treasure Island (FL): StatPearls Publishing. Available from https://www.ncbi.nlm.nih.gov/books/NBK545201/.

6. Jeukendrup, A. E., I. Rollo, and J. M. Carter. 2013. "Carbohydrate Mouth Rinse: Performance Effects and Mechanisms." December 2013. Retrieved from https://www.gssiweb.org/sports-science-exchange/article/sse-118-carbohydrate-mouth-rinse-performance-effects-and-mechanisms.

7. Mayer, E. A. 2018. *The Mind-Gut Connection: How the Hidden Conversation Within Our Bodies Impacts Our Mood, Our Choices, and Our Overall Health.* New York: Harper Wave.

8. Peirce, J. M. and K. Alviña. 2019. "The Role of Inflammation and the Gut Microbiome in Depression and Anxiety." *Journal of Neuroscience Research*, 97(10), 1223-1241. doi:10.1002/jnr.24476.

9. Spector, D. 2014. "An Evolutionary Explanation for Why We Crave Sugar." April 25, 2014. Retrieved December 24, 2020, from https://www.businessinsider.com/evolutionary-reason-we-love-sugar-2014-4.

10. Wu, Q. and X. Liang. 2018. "Food Therapy and Medical Diet Therapy of Traditional Chinese Medicine." *Clinical Nutrition Experimental* 18, 1–5. doi:10.1016/j.yclnex.2018.01.001.

2.4 Consider the Balance of Your Emotions

1. Barlow, D. H. 1988. *Anxiety and Its Disorders: The Nature and Treatment of Anxiety and Panic.* New York: The Guilford Press.

2. Chieng, R. 2020. "Ronny Chieng Thinks Amazon Prime Is Too Slow | Netflix Is a Joke." January 9, 2020. Retrieved January 10, 2021, from https://www.youtube.com/watch?v=BGEAiUeiaKs.

3. Chung, Y., J. Chen, and K. Ko. 2016. "Spleen Function and Anxiety in Chinese Medicine: A Western Medicine Perspective." *Chinese Medicine* 7, 110–123. doi: 10.4236/cm.2016.73012.

4. Gruber, J., I. B. Mauss, and M. Tamir. 2011. "A Dark Side of Happiness? How, When, and Why Happiness Is Not Always Good." *Perspectives on Psychological Science* 6(3), 222–233. doi:10.1177/1745691611406927.

5. Maciocia, G. 2005. *The Foundations of Chinese Medicine.* Edinburgh: Elsevier Churchill Livingstone.

6. Muzio, J. N. 2012. "The Optimism Bias: A Tour of the Irrationally Positive Brain." *Choice* 49(5), 908. Retrieved from http://eproxy.lib.hku.hk/login?url=https://www-proquest-com.eproxy.lib.hku.hk/trade-journals/optimism-bias-tour-irrationally-positive-brain/docview/921022521/se-2?accountid=14548.

7. Oishi, S., E. Diener, and R. E. Lucas. 2007. "The Optimum Level of Well-Being: Can People Be Too Happy?" *Perspectives on Psychological Science 2(4)*, 346–360. doi:10.1111/j.1745-6916.2007.00048.

8. Sugay, C. 2020. "Unhealthy Happiness: Its Underlit Dark Side and Negative Effects." October 17, 2020. Retrieved December 25, 2020, from https://positivepsychology.com/dark-side-of-happiness.

9. Weisinger, H. and J. P. Pawliw-Fry. 2016. *How to Perform Under Pressure: The Science of Doing Your Best When It Matters Most.* London: John Murray Learning.

10. Ye, J., S. Cai, W. M. Cheung, and H. W. Tsang. 2019. "An East Meets West Approach to the Understanding of Emotion Dysregulation in Depression: From Perspective to Scientific Evidence." *Frontiers in Psychology* 10. doi:10.3389/fpsyg.2019.00574.

2.5 Assess the Health of Your Fascia

1. Igarashi, G., C. Karashima, and M. Hoshiyama. 2015. "Effect of Cognitive Load on Seating Posture in Children." *Occupational Therapy International* 23(1), 48–56. doi:10.1002/oti.1405.

2. Michalak, J., J. Mischnat, and T. Teismann. 2014. "Sitting Posture Makes a Difference: Embodiment Effects on Depressive Memory Bias." *Clinical Psychology & Psychotherapy* 21(6), 519–524. https://doi.org/10.1002/cpp.1890.

3. Mikel, B. 2016. "Research Suggests Slouching Is Good for You (Sometimes)." April 7, 2016. Retrieved January 11, 2021, from https://www.inc.com/betsy-mikel/slouchers-rejoice-research-finds-perfect-posture-can-hinder-concentration.html.

4. Riskind, J. H. and C. C. Gotay. 1982. "Physical Posture: Could It Have Regulatory or Feedback Effects on Motivation and Emotion?" *Motivation and Emotion*, 6(3), 273–298. doi:10.1007/bf00992249.

5. Starrett, K., J. Starrett, and G. Cordoza. 2016. *Deskbound: Standing Up to a Sitting World.* Las Vegas: Victory Belt Publishing.

6. Tsay A., T. J. Allen, U. Proske, and M. J. Giummarra. 2015. "Sensing the

Body in Chronic Pain: A Review of Psychophysical Studies Implicating Altered Body Representation." *Neuroscience & Biobehavioral Reviews* 52, 221–232.

7. "Understanding the Stress Response." (n.d.). *Staying Healthy* (blog). Harvard Health Publishing. Retrieved January 15, 2021, from https://www.health.harvard.edu/staying-healthy/ understanding-the-stress-response.

8. Veenstra, L., I. K. Schneider, and S. L. Koole. 2017. "Embodied Mood Regulation: The Impact of Body Posture on Mood Recovery, Negative Thoughts, and Mood-Congruent Recall." *Cognition & Emotion* 31(7), 1361–1376. https://doi.org/10.1080/02699931.2016.1225003.

Part 3: Lifestyle Strategies for Dynamic Balance: Some Practical Pointers

3.1 Developing a Diet for Optimal Health and Performance

1. Beinfield, H. and E. Korngold. 1991. *Between Heaven and Earth: A Guide to Chinese Medicine.* New York: Random House Publishing Group.

2. Enders, C. 2015. "Why You Really Should (but Really Can't) Eat Horsemeat." January 9, 2015. Retrieved December 29, 2020, from https://www.theguardian.com/environment/2015/jan/09/ eating-wild-horsemeat-america.

3. Koliaki, C., T. Spinos, M. Spinou, M. Brinia, D. Mitsopoulou, and N. Katsilambros. 2018. "Defining the Optimal Dietary Approach for Safe, Effective and Sustainable Weight Loss in Overweight and Obese Adults." *Healthcare* 6(3), 73. doi:10.3390/healthcare6030073.

4. Ni, M. 1995. *The Yellow Emperor's Classic of Medicine.* Shambhala.

5. Parrella, N. 2020. "Good-for-You Foods: One Size Does Not Fit All." The Hill. March 12, 2020. Retrieved December 28, 2020, from https://thehill.com/opinion/ healthcare/487181-good-for-you-foods-one-size-does-not-fit-all.

6. Shuanlei T. and W. Qi. 2011. "Analysis of the Basic Principles of Dietary Regimen in Traditional Chinese Medicine." *Li Shi Zhen Chinese Medicine and Herbal* 22, 976–977.

7. Wongvibulsin, S. 2014. "Eat Right, Drink Well, Stress Less: Stress-Reducing Foods, Herbal Supplements, and Teas." Explore Integrative Medicine (blog), UCLA Health. Retrieved December 24, 2020, from https://exploreim.ucla.edu/nutrition/eat-right-drink-well-stress-less-stress-reducing-foods-herbal-supplements-and-teas.

8. Yue, X., L. Wang, D. Zhu, and Y. Zhou. 2018. *Basic Theory of Traditional Chinese Medicine.* Xinjiapo (Singapore): Nanyang chu ban she.

3.2 Mastering the Art of Breathing

1. Clark, M., S. Lucett, and B. G. Sutton. 2014. *NASM Essentials of Corrective Exercise Training.* Burlington, MA: Jones & Bartlett Learning.

2. Draeger-Muenke, R. and M. Muenke. 2012. "The Healing Energy of Breath in Traditional Chinese Medicine and Other Eastern Traditions." In Anbar, R.D. (ed.), "Functional Respiratory Disorders." *Respiratory Medicine.* Totowa, NJ: Humana Press.

3. HajGhanbari, B., C. Yamabayashi, T. R. Buna, J. D. Coelho, K. D. Freedman, T. A. Morton, W. D. Reid, et al. 2013. "Effects of Respiratory Muscle Training on Performance in Athletes." *Journal of Strength and Conditioning Research* 27(6), 1643–1663. doi:10.1519/jsc.0b013e318269f73f.

4. Hamasaki, H. 2020. "Effects of Diaphragmatic Breathing on Health: A Narrative Review." *Medicines* 7(10), 65. doi:10.3390/medicines7100065.

5. Zaccaro, A., A. Piarulli, M. Laurino, E. Garbella, D. Menicucci, B. Neri, and A. Gemignani. 2018. "How Breath-Control Can Change Your Life: A Systematic Review on Psycho-Physiological Correlates of Slow Breathing." *Frontiers in Human Neuroscience* 12, 353. https://doi.org/10.3389/fnhum.2018.00353.

3.3 Developing Harmony in Your Movement

1. Bartlett, R., J. Wheat, and M. Robins. 2007. "Is Movement Variability Important for Sports Biomechanists?" *Sports Biomechanics,* 6(2), 224–243. doi: 10.1080/14763140701322994.

2. Clark, M., S. Lucett, and B. G. Sutton. 2014. *NASM Essentials of Corrective Exercise Training.* Burlington, MA: Jones & Bartlett Learning.

3. Cook, G. 2017. *Movement: Functional Movement Systems: Screening, Assessment and Corrective Strategies.* Santa Cruz, CA: On Target Publications.

4. Dischiavi, S. L., A. A. Wright, E. J. Hegedus, and C. M. Bleakly. 2019. "Rethinking Dynamic Knee Valgus and Its Relation to Knee Injury: Normal Movement Requiring Control, Not Avoidance." *Journal of Orthopaedic & Sports Physical Therapy* 49, 216–218.

5. Kebaetse M., P. McClure, and N. A. Pratt. 1999. "Thoracic Position Effect on Shoulder Range of Motion, Strength, and Three-Dimensional Kinematics." *Archives of Physical Medicine and Rehabilitation* 80, 945–50.

6. Kroell, Jordan and Jonathan Mike. 2017. "Exploring the Standing Barbell Overhead Press." *Strength and Conditioning Journal* 39, 1. doi: 10.1519/ SSC.0000000000000324.

7. Manjunath Prasad, K. S., B. A. Gregson, G. Hargreaves, T. Byrnes, P. Winburn, and M. J. Matthews, Y. Mohamed, C. Doyle, and C. Thompson. 2016. "Quadrupedal Movement Training Improves Markers of Cognition and Joint Repositioning." *Human Movement Science* 47, 70–80. ISSN 0167-9457. https://doi.org/10.1016/j.humov.2016.02.002.

8. Mendelow, A. D. 2012. "Inversion Therapy in Patients with Pure Single Level Lumbar Discogenic Disease: A Pilot Randomized Trial." *Disability and Rehabilitation* 34(17), 1473–1480. doi: 10.3109/09638288.2011.647231.

9. Moreside, J. M. and S. M. McGill. 2012. "Hip Joint Range of Motion Improvements Using Three Different Interventions. *The Journal of Strength & Conditioning Research* 26(5), 1265–1273.

10. Myers, T. W. 2001. *Anatomy Trains: Myofascial Meridians for Manual and Movement Therapists.* Edinburgh: Churchill Livingstone.

11. Ng, B. H. and H. W. Tsang. 2009. "Psychophysiological Outcomes of Health Qigong for Chronic Conditions: A Systematic Review." *Psychophysiology* 46, 257–269.

12. Schleip, R. and D. G. Müller. 2013. "Training Principles for Fascial Connective Tissues: Scientific Foundation and Suggested Practical Applications." *Journal of Bodywork and Movement Therapies* 17(1) (January): 103–15. doi: 10.1016/j.jbmt.2012.06.007. Epub 2012 Jul 21. PMID: 23294691.

13. Starrett, K. and G. Cordoza. 2015. *Becoming a Supple Leopard: The Ultimate Guide to Resolving Pain, Preventing Injury, and Optimizing Athletic Performance.* Las Vegas, NV: Victory Belt Publishing.

14. Tubbs, R. S., S. Riech, K. Verma, J. Chern, M. Mortazavi, and A. Cohen-Gadol. 2011. "China's First Surgeon: Hua Tuo (c. 108–208 AD)." *Child's Nervous System*, Official Journal of the International Society for Pediatric Neurosurgery 27, 1357–60. doi: 10.1007/s00381-011-1423-z.

15. Wai, F. K. 2004. "On Hua Tuo's Position in the History of Chinese Medicine." *The American Journal of Chinese Medicine* 32(02), 313–320. doi: 10.1142/s0192415x04001965.

3.4 Incorporating TCM Recovery Tools

1. Akbari, A., S. M. Zadeh, M. Ramezani, and S. M. S. Zadeh. 2013. "The Effect of Hijama (Cupping) on Oxidative Stress Indexes & Various Blood Factors in Patients Suffering from Diabetes Type II." *Switzerland Research Park Journal* 102, 9.

2. Al-Bedah, A. M., I. S. Elsubai, N. A. Qureshi, T. S. Aboushanab, G. I. Ali, A. T. El-Olemy, M. S. Alqaed, et al. 2019. "The Medical Perspective of Cupping Therapy: Effects and Mechanisms of Action." *Journal of Traditional and Complementary Medicine* 9(2), 90–97. doi:10.1016/j.jtcme.2018.03.003.

3. Cao, H. 2010. "Clinical Research Evidence of Cupping Therapy in China: A Systematic Literature Review." *BMC Complementary and Alternative Medicine* 10, 70.

4. Cheatham, S. W., E. Kreiswirth, and R. Baker. 2019. "Does a Light Pressure Instrument Assisted Soft Tissue Mobilization Technique Modulate Tactile Discrimination and Perceived Pain in Healthy Individuals with DOMS?" *The Journal of the Canadian Chiropractic Association* 63(1), 18–25.

5. Cheatham, S. W., R. Baker, and E. Kreiswirth. 2019. "Instrument Assisted Soft-Tissue Mobilization: A Commentary on Clinical Practice Guidelines for Rehabilitation Professionals." *International Journal of Sports Physical Therapy* 14(4), 670–682. Retrieved from https://pubmed.ncbi. nlm.nih.gov/31440416.

6. Kim, J. I., M. S. Lee, D. H. Lee, K. Boddy, and E. Ernst. 2011. "Cupping for Treating Pain: A Systematic Review." *Evidence-Based Complementary and Alternative Medicine.*

7. Marion, T., K. Cao, and J. Roman. 2018. "Gua Sha, or Coining Therapy." *JAMA Dermatology* 154(7), 788. https://doi.org/10.1001/ jamadermatol.2018.0615.

8. Moncada, S., R. M. Palmer, and E. A. Higgs. 1991. "Nitric Oxide: Physiology, Pathophysiology, and Pharmacology. *Pharmacology* 43, 109–142.

9. Nazari, G., P. Bobos, J. C. MacDermid, and T. Birmingham. 2019. "The Effectiveness of Instrument-Assisted Soft Tissue Mobilization in Athletes, Participants Without Extremity or Spinal Conditions, and Individuals with Upper Extremity, Lower Extremity, and Spinal Conditions: A Systematic Review." *Archives of Physical Medicine and Rehabilitation* 100(9), 1726–1751. https://doi.org/10.1016/j. apmr.2019.01.017.

10. Nielsen, A., B. Kligler, and B. S. Koll. 2012. "Safety Protocols for Gua Sha (Press-Stroking) and Baguan (Cupping)." *Complementary Therapies in Medicine*, 20(5), 340–344. https://doi.org/10.1016/j.ctim.2012.05.004.

11. Tang, K. W. 2020. *Gua Sha: An Ancient Therapy for Contemporary Illnesses.* Hackensack, NJ: World Scientific.

Part 3 Debrief: To Your Good Health

1. Davies, K. J. 2016. "Adaptive Homeostasis." *Molecular Aspects of Medicine* 49 (June), 1–7. [PMC free article] [PubMed].

2. Wang, Y. 2019. "The Scientific Nature of Traditional Chinese Medicine in the Post-Modern Era." *Journal of Traditional Chinese Medical Sciences* 6(3), 195–200. doi:10.1016/j.jtcms.2019.09.003.

MERIDIANS AND QI

The meridians are pathways where Qi and blood are circulated. Each of the 12 Meridians has physiological functions that are vital to human health and performance. Ancient physicians outlined how each pathway is connected to a Zang-Fu (organ) and its significance in illness. As a reminder, Yin meridians are the ones in the front side of the body, and Yang are the ones in the back. Also recall the highway example from Chapter 1.3 that illustrates how the ideal amount of Qi is like traffic that is smooth and unobstructed and not going too fast over the speed limit.

Hand				
Distribution	**Meridian**	**Significance in Treatments**		
Yin: starts from the chest, runs along the front arm to the hand	Lung Meridian of Hand	Lung and throat diseases		Chest-related diseases
	Pericardium Meridian of Hand	Heart and stomach diseases	Psychotic diseases	
	Heart Meridian of Hand	Heart diseases		
Yang: starts from the hand, runs along the back arm to the head	Large Intestine Meridian of Hand	Forehead, oronasal, dental diseases		Throat diseases, hot/fevers
	Triple Burner Meridian of Hand	Diseases on the lateral sides of the head and torso, along the rib cage	Ophthalmic and ear diseases	
	Small Intestine Meridian of Hand	Back of the head and scapula, and psychotic diseases		

Foot		
Distribution	**Meridian**	**Significance in Treatment**
Yang: starts from the head, runs across the trunk and along the front, lateral, and back sides of the leg to the foot	Stomach Meridian of Foot	Forehead, mouth, throat, and spleen
	Gallbladder Meridian of Foot	Both sides of the head, the ears, and lateral sides of the torso and rib cage
	Bladder Meridian of Foot	Back of the head, lower back, and waist
Yin: starts from the foot, runs along the inner side of the leg, crosses the chest and abdomen to the head	Spleen Meridian of Foot	Spleen and stomach diseases
	Liver Meridian of Foot	Liver diseases
	Kidney Meridian of Foot	Kidney, lung, and throat diseases

FASCIAL MERIDIANS

The fitness world often talks about the twelve fascial meridians identified by Thomas Myers in his bestselling book *Anatomy Trains*, as listed below.

- Superficial Back Line
- Superficial Front Line
- Lateral Line (two sides)
- Spiral Line
- Superficial Arm Line
- Deep Back Arm Line
- Deep Front Arm Line
- Superficial Back Arm Line
- Back Functional Line
- Front Functional Line
- Ipsilateral Functional Line
- Deep Front Line

These twelve fascial meridians have fundamentally changed the way we look at movement. That is, instead of zooming into an isolated muscle, we look at how a group of muscles must work together synergistically to produce silky and elegant movements.

The most common condition we see, whether in athletes or non-athletes, is a hunched position where the front lines have adapted to be shorter than usual and the back lines are longer than usual, typically caused by either prolonged sitting or from being in stressful situations (as a protective mechanism). If this is the case for you or an athlete you are coaching, a sensible plan is to work on exercises that shorten the back lines (exercises such as the deadlift) and incorporate techniques that lengthen the front lines (the Bear chest opening movement, massage, cupping, and Gua Sha that targets different areas of the front lines), before doing the Tiger as a way for the brain to relearn the dynamic relationship between the front and back lines. Again, in an ideal world, the front and back lines should be able to dynamically lengthen and shorten depending on the task at hand.

FOODS

Use the tables in this Appendix to help you analyze your diet.

1. Flavors: Too Much, Too Little, Just Right

In keeping with the theme of this book, the challenge for each of us is to maintain a balance of flavors in our diet. The following table summarizes how having the right amount of each flavor can help our bodies cope not just with athletic performance but with everything that happens in life. In Appendix D, we'll go into more detail about how you can analyze your own diet and adjust the flavor balance to suit your body constitution, season, and so on.

BALANCING FLAVOR IN OUR DIET

Flavor	Too Little	Right Amount	Too Much
Sour	The liver Qi is not nourished and retained, causing a divergence of the liver Qi. Too little sour flavor manifests as grumpiness, irritation, and annoyance (e.g., pregnancy cravings for sour foods).	Sour foods can help digestion by counteracting the effects of fatty foods. The sour flavor has retaining properties, so it also helps to retain liver Qi and avoid excessive divergence. This is also why sour drinks are more popular in hotter regions like Southeast Asia.	Too much of the sour flavor may interfere with digestion, thereby creating stagnant energy (accumulating dampness).
Sweet	The spleen Qi becomes weak and may lead to a bloated feeling and a lack of energy (e.g., some people who menstruate may crave sugar prior to their cycle, or children who are at the stage of developing spleen [TCM] may have stronger cravings for sweets).	Sweet is the most common flavor and forms the center of our diet. It harmonizes well with the other flavors. It stimulates circulation, thereby giving us energy. Sweet flavor also acts as a lubricant for dryness.	Too much sweetness is tough for the spleen and gut to digest. It can lead to the formation of phlegm and heat, making one feel lethargic.
Bitter	Too little bitter flavor manifests as annoyance, irritation, and headaches, especially in the summer.	The bitter flavor stimulates digestion and clears out dampness and heat. The Chinese have also used it to fight inflammation and induce bowel movements.	It can injure the spleen and stomach digestive functions. Bitter flavor is like an axe, as it expels waste (e.g., excessive heat, dampness) in the body. But excessive use harms our normal systems and expels our healthy Qi (e.g., nausea or vomiting from antibiotics).

Flavor	Too Little	Right Amount	Too Much
Spicy	Too little spicy flavor manifests as greater aversion to cold. It also weakens the immune system, making it easier to catch a cold.	The spicy flavor removes stagnation and encourages Qi-blood circulation. It warms the body and stimulates digestion, which is why eating spicy foods during the winter is especially helpful (e.g., mulled wine).	Too much spicy flavor overstimulates Qi and blood, which ultimately depletes or expels the fluids and energy in the body. Fingernails and toenails may become brittle, since there isn't enough water left inside to moisturize and nourish them.
Salty	Too little salty flavor may result in diarrhea, muscle weakness, frequent urination, and so on. It may also cause the body to be unable to retain sufficient water and fluids.	Vital to human health, the salty flavor regulates the moisture balance in the body, stimulates digestive function, and improves concentration.	In Western medicine, the kidneys are in charge of regulating the sodium and potassium balance. In TCM, too much salt causes an excess in the kidney Qi (water phase) and affects a person's heart Qi (fire phase), causing one to experience fatigue or even heart failure—which is similar to Western medicine's understanding of excess consumption of sodium.

2. Nature of Selected Foods

FRUITS

Fruit	Nature
Almond	Warm
Apple	Cold
Banana	Cool
Coconut	Neutral
Grapes	Neutral
Guava	Warm
Hazelnut	Neutral
Lemon	Neutral
Lychee	Warm
Mango	Cool
Olive	Neutral
Orange	Cold
Papaya	Neutral
Peach	Neutral
Pineapple	Neutral
Pomelo	Cool
Strawberry	Cold
Tomato	Slightly Cool
Watermelon	Cold

VEGETABLES

Vegetable	Nature
Bitter Cucumber	Cool
Black Fungus	Neutral
Cabbage	Cold
Carrot	Neutral
Chili Pepper	Hot
Chinese Cabbage	Neutral
Coriander	Warm
Cucumber	Cool
Eggplant	Cold
Garlic	Warm
Ginger	Warm
Green Onion	Warm
Mushroom	Neutral
Onion	Neutral
Pumpkin	Warm
Radish	Cold
Spinach	Cold
Taro	Neutral

GRAINS AND BEANS

Grain or Bean	Nature
Barley	Cool
Black Beans	Neutral
Corn	Cool
Green Beans	Neutral
Lentils	Neutral
Malt	Slightly Warm
Oat	Neutral
Peas	Neutral
Potato	Neutral
Soy Beans	Neutral
Sweet Potato	Neutral
Tofu	Cool
Wheat	Cool

SEAFOOD

Seafood	Nature
Abalone	Neutral
Clam	Cold
Crab	Cold
Eel	Warm
Most Fish	Neutral
Octopus	Neutral
Seaweed	Cold
Shrimp	Warm

MEAT

Meat	Nature
Beef	Neutral
Chicken	Warm
Chicken Egg	Neutral
Deer	Warm
Duck Egg	Cold
Goose	Warm
Horse	Cold
Lamb	Warm
Pork	Neutral
Rabbit	Cold
Wild Boar	Neutral

DRINKS

Drink	Nature	Flavor
Beer	Cool	Sweet, Bitter
Cacao	Warm	Bitter
Coffee	Warm	Sweet, Bitter
Cow's Milk	Neutral	Sweet
Honey	Neutral	Sweet
Jasmine	Warm	Sweet, Spicy
Liquor	Warm	Varies
Peppermint	Cold	Sweet, Bitter
Rose	Warm	Sweet, Bitter
Soy Milk	Neutral	Sweet
Wine	Warm	Sweet, Spicy

3. Seasonal Food Tips

SPRING

Spring is a time of rebirth, renewal, and growth.

- Increase the amounts of nutritious foods to boost the immune system.
- Avoid foods that are cool in nature, and minimize foods that are hot, such as chili.
- Take advantage of the diverse range of available fruits and vegetables during this season.

SUMMER

Summer is hot and dry or humid depending on the geographical location. The best foods for summer are cooling and hydrating.

- Avoid overeating and use less seasoning to protect the digestive organs (spleen and stomach).
- Eat sweet- and sour-flavored foods (as in sweet *and* sour, not sweet *or* sour) that are cool or neutral in nature.
- Eat sweet foods that stimulate body fluids (e.g., spinach, watermelon, orange, tofu, goose, chicken, apple, cow's milk, grapes).
- Eat bitter foods that help expel excessive heat and dampness.

AUTUMN

Autumn is a season of transition. Focus on eating foods that prepare the body for winter.

- Eat more spicy flavors (but not too much) to stimulate liver Qi.
- For those with Yin deficiencies, consume spicy foods that are cool in nature.
- For those with Yang deficiencies, consume spicy foods that are warm in nature.
- Eat ginger, leeks, cinnamon, garlic, and radishes to nourish the lungs.
- Eat quinoa, rice, and oats for this transitional season, as mildly sweet foods improve energy in the spleen.

WINTER

Winter is a season of rest, so focus on eating foods that are cooked and warm in nature.

- Avoid foods that are cold in nature, especially salad and raw food.
- Eat foods that nourish the kidneys, such as black beans and lentils.

4. Herbal Teas

Instead of drinking three to four cups of coffee, which amp you up, here are some alternatives that do the opposite—calm you down. The following herbs and teas are commonly used for their calming effect and to reduce stress-related insomnia, anxiety, or anger.

- **Chamomile** is a popular herb that is often used to relieve stress-induced symptoms, such as insomnia and digestive system disorders.

- **Mint** also is commonly used to relieve stress. Its spicy and cooling properties are associated with the lung and liver meridians, and it is used to expel wind heat, relieve headache, relieve sore throat, and soothe anxiety and stress by clearing liver Qi stagnation.

- **Barley tea** is known for its ability to detoxify deficient Qi, blood, and Yin. It does that by regulating the stomach while stimulating blood and body fluids. It is also a great choice for diabetics because of its ability to strengthen the spleen and pancreas (Zang-Fu).

- **Passionflower** is a cooling and bitter herb marketed for its ability to treat sleep disorders, nervous tension, and anxiety. Passionflower in TCM is associated with the heart and liver meridians. It can also help cool and stabilize those with excessive Yang energy.

DIET GUIDELINES FOR DIFFERENT CONSTITUTIONS

The following tables provide suggestions for foods that you should consider adding to or deleting from your diet based on your body constitution type. These are not exhaustive lists.

Qi Deficiency

Eat foods that nourish the spleen and the gut.

Eat to Heal	
✗ **Avoid**	✓ **Emphasize**
Fried or salty food	Easily digestible foods
Iced foods or drinks	Food more balanced food in nature
Refined sugar	Strive for variety of foods
Refined grains	Corn
Beer	Chestnut
Dairy	Mushroom
	Chicken
	Fish
	Lentils
	Quinoa
	Oats
	Pumpkin
	Sweet Potato

Yang Deficiency

Eat foods that are neutral, warm, and nourishing.

Eat to Heal	
✗ Avoid	✓ Emphasize
Foods cool in nature Iced foods or drinks	Foods warm in nature Beef Lamb Shrimp Legumes Pumpkin Ginger Chestnuts Wheat

Yin Deficiency

Eat foods to clear deficient heat. Avoid stimulating foods and drinks.

Eat to Heal	
✗ Avoid	✓ Emphasize
Refined sugar Spicy foods Refined protein Food and drinks hot in nature Caffeine	Cooling foods Foods with bitter flavor Spinach Celery Wheat Banana Watermelon Tofu Honey Coconut water

Phlegm-Wetness

Eat foods to nourish the spleen and to clear phlegm and dampness. Avoid raw, cold, oily, and heavily processed foods.

Eat to Heal	
✗ Avoid	✓ Emphasize
Dairy Fatty grains Refined wheat products Deep-fried food Sugar and sweeteners	Celery Spinach Mushrooms Almonds Walnuts Black tea Garlic

Wetness-Heat

Eat nourishing foods to clear heat.

Eat to Heal	
✗ Avoid	✓ Emphasize
Lamb Ginger Chili peppers	Celery Oats Nuts Beans Cabbage Watermelon

Blood Stasis

Eat foods that stimulate blood.

Eat to Heal	
✗ Avoid	**✓ Emphasize**
Refined grains Fried foods	Pork liver Grapes Spinach Carrots Hazelnuts Chicken Lamb

Qi Stagnation

Eat foods that stimulate Qi.

Eat to Heal	
✗ Avoid	**✓ Emphasize**
Refined grains Sugar Fried foods Keto diet	Onion Garlic Cabbage Broccoli Mustard greens Kale Radish Basil Fennel Mint Grapefruit Green apples

THE BEN CASE STUDY AND ANALYSIS

In Part 2, the Ben case study provided examples used to help illustrate how to use and interpret the constitution questionnaire and identify potential imbalances in diet, emotions, and fascia. Here are the details of the analysis not included in the Part 2 chapters.

1. Background

Ben is a thirty-three-year-old investment banker from San Francisco. He is 5 feet, 11 inches tall and slender. Outside of his stressful work, he enjoys working out and playing basketball. Although Ben is not an elite athlete, his competitive spirit is second to none. Because of that, he has studied numerous books and internet videos on performance enhancement. In the spring of 2019, he decided to hire a personal trainer to help him reach his goals. He also decided to document his daily routine and workout progress on Instagram.

After three months on a strict diet and workout regimen, here were Ben's results:

BEN'S PROGRESS

	Weight	Squat 1RM	Deadlift 1RM	Bench Press 1RM
Start	164 lb.	100 kg	130 kg	60 kg
End	175 lb.	115 kg	150 kg	70 kg
Gain	+11 lb.	+15 kg	+20 kg	+10 kg

However, Ben felt sluggish and tired, so obviously something about his new plan wasn't working for him.

To analyze Ben's constitution and potential imbalances, we needed to know the following details as well—season, geographical location, climate—to examine whether he was eating in accordance with the surrounding environment.

What is the current season?	Spring
Which city/town are you in?	San Francisco
What is the climate?	The temperature is in the mid-70s (about 23 degrees Celsius). Humidity around 80%.

2. Analysis of Ben's Constitution

Ben completed the body constitution questionnaire (see Chapter 2.1). Here is the complete table followed by a summary of his results.

QI DEFICIENCY

	Never	Seldom	Sometimes	Frequent	Always
Fatigued	1	2	3	(4)	5
Shortness of breath/panting (compared to people of your age)	1	(2)	3	4	5
Heart palpitations	(1)	2	3	4	5
Dizzy or lightheaded	1	2	(3)	4	5
Frequent colds and flu (especially when season changes)	(1)	2	3	4	5
Aloof and emotionally distant	(1)	2	3	4	5
Weak, breathy, or feeble voice	(1)	2	3	4	5
Excessive perspiration or night sweats	1	(2)	3	4	5
Total score divided by 8: 1.875					

YANG DEFICIENCY

	Never	Seldom	Sometimes	Frequent	Always
Cold hands and feet/pale skin	(1)	2	3	4	5
Cold intolerance (sensitive to cold environments)	(1)	2	3	4	5
More layers of clothing than those around you	(1)	2	3	4	5
Chills in the abdomen, lower back, or knees	(1)	2	3	4	5
Prone to sickness/getting sick all the time (weak immune system)	(1)	2	3	4	5
Erectile dysfunction (male) or loss of sex drive (male or female)	(1)	2	3	4	5
Stomachache or diarrhea after eating cold/raw food and beverages	1	2	(3)	4	5
Repressed	(1)	2	3	4	5
Total score divided by 8: 1.25					

YIN DEFICIENCY

	Never	Seldom	Sometimes	Frequent	Always
Warm or burning sensations in hands and feet (like to expose limbs or touch cool surfaces)	1	(2)	3	4	5
Feeling hot but no fever	1	2	3	(4)	5
Dry skin/cracked lips	1	(2)	3	4	5
Dark/burgundy-colored lips (natural state without makeup)	1	(2)	3	4	5
Constipation/dry hard stool	1	2	3	4	(5)
Redness/flushing of cheeks or face	1	2	(3)	4	5
Dry eyes	1	(2)	3	4	5
Dry mouth or constant thirst	1	2	3	4	(5)
Total score divided by 8: 3.125					

PHLEGM-WETNESS

	Never	Seldom	Sometimes	Frequent	Always
Chest tightness/ abdominal bloating	1	2	(3)	4	5
Heaviness in limbs and body/lethargic	1	2	3	4	(5)
Delayed or slow bowel movements	1	2	3	4	(5)
Oily forehead	1	2	(3)	4	5
Puffy eyes	(1)	2	3	4	5
Mouth feels sticky	(1)	2	3	4	5
Excessive mucus in throat	(1)	2	3	4	5
Thick tongue coating	1	2	(3)	4	5
Total score divided by 8: 2.75					

WETNESS-HEAT

	Never	Seldom	Sometimes	Frequent	Always
Oily face/nose	1	2	3	4	(5)
Prone to acne	1	2	3	4	(5)
Bitter/bad taste in mouth	1	(2)	3	4	5
Sticky stool/tenesmus (sensation of needing to pass stool)	1	2	3	(4)	5
Hot or burning urine/dark urine (dark like amber)	(1)	2	3	4	5
Yellow discharge (female only)	1	2	3	4	5
Sweaty testicles (male only)	1	2	(3)	4	5
Total score divided by 6: 3.333					

BLOOD STASIS

	Never	Seldom	Sometimes	Frequent	Always
Petechiae/ecchymosis (unexplained bruising without bumping into things)	(1)	2	3	4	5
Rashes on face	1	(2)	3	4	5
Body aches	1	2	3	(4)	5
Dull skin tone	1	(2)	3	4	5
Dark circles under the eyes	1	2	3	4	(5)
Poor memory/forgetfulness	1	2	3	(4)	5
Dark red or purple lips (natural state without makeup)	(1)	2	3	4	5
Total score divided by 7: 2.714					

QI STAGNATION

	Never	Seldom	Sometimes	Frequent	Always
Depressed or unmotivated	(1)	2	3	4	5
Anxiety/frustration	1	(2)	3	4	5
Emotional and sensitive	1	(2)	3	4	5
Easily frightened/fearful	(1)	2	3	4	5
Mastalgia (breast pain for women)/ discomfort around the sides of rib cage (both men and women)	(1)	2	3	4	5
Sighing	1	(2)	3	4	5
Sensation of lump in the throat	(1)	2	3	4	5
Total score divided by 7: 1.429					

BALANCED HEALTH

	Never	Seldom	Sometimes	Frequent	Always
Easily fatigued	5	4	(3)	2	1
Weak/breathy voice	5	4	3	2	(1)
Constantly feeling down or gloomy	5	4	3	(2)	1
Cold aversion (including to AC or fans in summer)	5	4	3	2	(1)
Sensitive to natural changes in the environment (climate, weather)	5	(4)	3	2	1
Insomnia	5	4	3	(2)	1
Forgetful	5	(4)	3	2	1
Total score divided by 7: 2.43					

Constitution	Ben's Numbers
Qi Deficiency	1.875
Yang Deficiency	1.25
Yin Deficiency	3.125
Phlegm-Wetness	2.75
Wetness-Heat	3.333
Blood Stasis	2.714
Qi Stagnation	1.429
Balanced Health	2.43

3. Analysis of Ben's Diet

For three days, Ben documented what he ate and drank. His target was at least 3,000 calories. He then used the information in Appendix C to identify the flavors and natures of the food he consumed. The first tables outline his diet, followed by a summary analysis of the flavors and natures in the foods he ate.

DAY 1

Time	Name and portion of food/drink (roughly)	Flavor(s)	Nature
7:30 a.m.	4-egg omelet with spinach and cheese	Sweet	Eggs: Neutral Spinach: Cool Cheese: Neutral in small quantities
	1 bagel	Sweet	Warm
	1 cup of whole cow's milk	Sweet	Neutral
9:00 a.m.	Iced coffee	Bitter	Warm*
10:00 a.m.	Mass-gainer shake	Sweet	Hot
12:30 p.m.	Pan-fried double chicken breast	Sweet, Salty	Warm
	Boiled broccoli with salt	Sweet, Salty	Cool
	Brown rice	Sweet	Neutral
	Coffee	Bitter	Warm
3:00 p.m.	Roasted mixed nuts	Salty, Sweet	Hot
	Banana	Sweet	Neutral
5:00 p.m.	Pan-fried small chicken breast	Sweet, Salty	Warm
	Boiled broccoli with salt	Sweet, Salty	Cool
	Brown rice	Sweet	Neutral
7:00 p.m.	Pan-fried sirloin steak	Sweet, Salty	Warm
	Stir-fried spinach	Sweet, Salty	Cool
	Baked Potato	Sweet	Neutral
9:30 p.m.	Casein protein shake	Sweet	Hot
	1 cup of whole cow's milk	Sweet	Neutral

*Coffee is cool in nature, as it is a fruit. However, the property of the fruit is changed after roasting. It is also worth noting that coffee is four thousand years younger than Chinese medicine, so the effects of coffee are not recorded in ancient texts.

DAY 2

Time	Name and portion of food/drink (roughly)	Flavor(s)	Nature
8:00 a.m.	Sausage, egg, and cheese bagel	Salty, Sweet	Pan-fried sausage: Hot Egg: Neutral Cheese: Neutral Bagel: Warm
	1 large latte	Bitter, Sweet	Milk: Neutral Coffee: Warm
10:00 a.m.	Mass-gainer shake	Sweet	Hot
12:30 p.m.	Pan-fried double chicken breast	Salty, Sweet	Warm
	Boiled broccoli with salt	Salty, Sweet	Cool
	Brown rice	Sweet	Neutral
	Iced black coffee	Bitter	Warm
3:00 p.m.	Roasted mixed nuts	Salty, Sweet	Warm
	Banana	Sweet	Neutral
4:00 p.m.	Pan-fried small chicken breast	Salty, Sweet	Warm
	Boiled broccoli with salt	Salty, Sweet	Cool
	Brown rice	Sweet	Neutral
7:00 p.m.	Pan-fried sirloin steak	Salty, Sweet	Warm
	Stir-fried green beans	Salty, Sweet	Cool
	Baked potato	Salty, Sweet	Neutral
9:30 p.m.	Casein protein shake	Sweet	Hot
	1 cup of whole cow's milk	Sweet	Neutral

DAY 3			
Time	**Name and portion of food/drink (roughly)**	**Flavor(s)**	**Nature**
8:00 a.m.	Bacon, egg, and cheese bagel	Salty, Sweet	Pan-fried bacon: Hot Egg: Neutral Cheese: Neutral Bagel: Warm
	1 large latte	Bitter, Sweet	Milk: Neutral Coffee: Warm
10:00 a.m.	Mass-gainer shake	Sweet	Hot
12:30 p.m.	Pan-fried double chicken breast	Salty, Sweet	Warm
	Boiled broccoli with salt	Salty	Cool
	Baked potato	Salty, Sweet	Neutral
	Iced black coffee	Bitter	Warm
3:00 p.m.	Banana and peanut butter sandwich with wheat bread	Sweet, Salty	Banana: Neutral Peanut butter: Warm Wheat bread: Neutral
5:00 p.m.	Mixed nuts	Salty, Sweet	Hot
7:30 p.m.	Chicken burrito with medium spicy salsa	Salty, Sweet, Spicy	Chicken: Warm Tortilla wrap and rice: Neutral Lettuce and tomato: Cool
	Salad with minimal dressing	Sweet	Cool
	Chips and guacamole	Salty, Sweet, Sour	Chips: Hot Guacamole: Cool
9:30 p.m.	Casein protein shake	Sweet	Hot
	1 cup whole cow's milk	Sweet	Neutral

Ben then added up how often the different flavors and natures appeared in his diet and came up with the results shown in the following table.

SUMMARY ANALYSIS OF BEN'S DIET

| | FLAVOR | | | | | NATURE | | | | |
| | | | | | | Yin ⟵—————————⟶ Yang | | | | |
	Sour	Sweet	Bitter	Spicy	Salty	Cold	Cool	Neutral	Warm	Hot
Day 1	0	17	2	0	7	0	4	8	6	3
Day 2	0	14	2	0	9	0	3	8	7	3
Day 3	0	12	2	0	8	0	4	8	6	5
TOTAL	0	43	6	0	24	0	11	24	19	11

From these numbers, we can conclude the following:

- The nature of Ben's food indicates a Yin deficiency (no cold and relatively few cool foods compared to warm and hot ones). This could explain why Ben feels hot, is constipated, and is constantly thirsty.

- The flavors indicate wetness-heat (because of the heavy emphasis on sweet flavors). This contributes to why Ben feels bloated and lethargic, has slow bowel movements, and is prone to acne.

ACKNOWLEDGMENTS

W riting a book has been one of the toughest—yet most rewarding—tasks that we've ever attempted. We worked closely with people around the globe and in different time zones, which sometimes made it challenging to further develop and fine-tune our manuscript. We're profoundly grateful to many people for helping us throughout the publishing process. And really, writing this book has only deepened our appreciation for the collective effort that a finished product represents.

Warmest thanks are due to Greenleaf Book Group for realizing our book-writing dream. Thank you to our developmental editor, Sue Reynard, for miraculously transforming our messy first draft into a tight and readable manuscript. Sue is truly a special talent! Thank you to our executive editor, Jessica Choi, for your calming and encouraging words throughout the editing process. We also thank our project manager, Lindsay Bohls, for connecting us to the right people at various stages of this publishing process. Thank you to our consultant, Danny Sandoval, for the initial tips and guidance before we buckled down and put in the hard work. Thank you to our designer, Mimi Bark, for the beautiful book cover, and layout designer, Brian Phillips, for the interior page-designs. We're grateful also to designers Neil Gonzalez, Chase Quarterman, Laurie MacQueen, and Stewart Cundy for their work on the book. Warmest thanks are extended to editors Judy Marchman, Kirstin Andrews, and Tonya Trybula for their valuable input throughout the various stages of the editing process. Many thanks to Senior

Marketing Strategist, Chelsea Richards, and also Distribution Account Coordinator, Tiffany Barrientos, for helping us get this book out into the world.

We would like to extend a special thanks to the team at StevenC Photography, photographer Steven Chui and assistants Jac and Shawn, for the amazing photos. Not only was the photo shoot a blast, but Steven also ensured that the shot angles really captured the essence of the moves we were demonstrating.

From Andy

My wife has played every role that a person can imagine: spouse, best friend, cheerleader, critic, designer, editor, listener, and counselor. This book could not have been completed without her. Alison, thank you so much for your support. Like everything else in life, we conquered it together!

To my dad, C. C. Chan; my mom, Salina Fung; and my brother, Kenny Chan, thank you for the unconditional support for all that I do.

To my in-laws, C. W. Chiu and Teresa Ho, thank you for your precious advice and input throughout the writing process.

Enormous gratitude is extended to Amy Acuff, Dr. Eduardo Santos, and Dr. Ronald Wagner for endorsing *Dynamic Balance*. You guys are the model professionals that I look up to; having your endorsements is truly something I am proud about and grateful for.

Special shoutout to the best hairstylist in Hong Kong, Fernando Viseu, for ensuring that I look my best for all my major life events.

Thank you, Mr. Tommy Adams, for believing in me back in my high school days. What a blessing it was to have someone who believed in me and defended me when others doubted. Mr. Adams, I hope this book makes you proud!

Thank you, coach Arturo Solís, for instilling in me the mindset when I was an 11th grader that talent without hard work, dedication, and commitment is a wasted talent.

I am forever indebted to my second family at Optimum Performance Studio—Kevin Rushton, Phoebe Ho, Raymond Ng, Wayne Clark, Edwin Teunissen, Lolita, and Sharon, thank you for all the opportunities, patience, guidance, tough love, and support over the years. It would be impossible to count all the ways that you all have helped me in my career.

My journey as a fitness instructor has been a blast. I am grateful for the fact that I can always have Annabelle Tsang and Ying Yee Chan to count on no matter how challenging and obscure the projects are. Annabelle, thank you for your assistance with many of my public speaking gigs and also your willingness to step in on short notice for the photo shoot for the book; you were a great model of Dynamic Balance. Ying Yee, I truly appreciate all your behind-the-scenes support.

To my mentors, Emily Tan, Ross Eathorne, Audrey Lo, Derek Poon, Alex Poole, and Ryan Charem, thank you for being great role models and offering the constructive feedback that has made me a better coach and presenter.

To my friends Jacky Ma, Nikki Cheung, Sharon Kao, Amanda Niem, Josh Ho, and Carl Au, thank you for always lending an ear and the practical wisdom on those frustrating days when I felt stuck. Being able to talk you guys on a regularly basis is gratifying yet humbling—gratifying because you all are willing to point out ways that I could improve in, humbling because you all are so wise and intelligent!

There are several people that I have learned so much from that their names must be recognized. Kelly Starrett, Stuart McGill, Thomas Myers, Robert Schleip, Gray Cook, Gary Gray. They and other great researchers, allied health professionals, and coaches have influenced my thoughts in many ways. Their work and ideas have been sprinkled throughout the book and are the cornerstone of an exercise regime that empowers humans to move freely as we are designed.

From Stella

Mom, thank you for your unconditional love and support over the years.

I would like to express my deep gratitude to my mentor in Taiwan, Dr. Liong-Chuan Lin, a.k.a. "Shifu." Your teachings have enlightened me to see Chinese medicine from a whole new perspective and gave me so much inspiration when I was writing this book.

ABOUT THE AUTHORS

Tsz Chiu "Andy" Chan, MS, CSCS

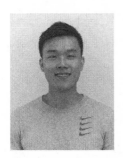

Andy is a certified strength and conditioning specialist, educator, and presenter from Hong Kong. With a master's degree in exercise science, Andy has a genuine passion for making a positive impact in the fitness industry through learning and sharing different unique methodologies. He currently teaches education courses on behalf of companies such as the National Academy of Sports Medicine, TRX, TriggerPoint Performance, and Power Plate. As a presenter, he has made guest appearances in Hong Kong television shows, as well as presenting at different public fitness events.

Yat Kwan "Stella" Wong, PhD

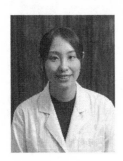

Being a second-generation traditional Chinese medicine (TCM) physician in her family, Stella was inspired by her mother to pursue the best TCM training programs. Stella obtained her undergraduate degree from Beijing University of Chinese Medicine. She is a licensed TCM practitioner in Hong Kong and obtained her PhD in

Chinese medicine from the University of Hong Kong, specializing in acupuncture and mental health disorders. She has also learned from experts in the field, such as Lin's Orthopaedics, and in areas such as scalp acupuncture and sinew acupuncture.